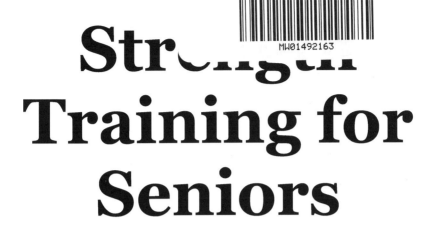

Strength Training for Seniors

Build Muscle and Increase Mobility With a 12-Week Workout Plan

Jade K. Miles

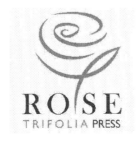

ROSE
TRIFOLIA PRESS

ISBN: Print 978-1-955661-01-0
        Ebook 978-1-955661-02-7

Table of Contents

SPECIAL BONUS

Want this Bonus Book for <u>FREE</u>?

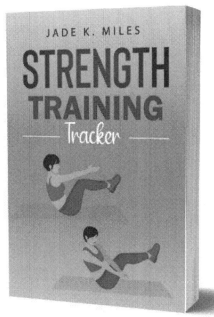

Get <u>FREE</u>, unlimited access to it and all of my new books by joining my Fan Base!

Scan with your camera to join!

Who Is the Author?

Hi, I'm Jade.

I'm a fitness coach and personal trainer with over 20 years of experience in the industry.

I'm on a mission to guide people through their fitness journey to become the best versions of themselves. I want to help people improve their health and find happiness through living a healthy lifestyle.

I believe an active lifestyle is more than just what exercise you do. I think it's a combination of exercise, nutrition, and lifestyle that contribute to a healthy life.

Why Was This Book Written?

Throughout my career, I have witnessed first-hand the barriers that prevent people from living a healthy lifestyle. The main thing I've noticed is people start to become more sedentary with age.

Aware of the dangers a sedentary lifestyle had on seniors, I knew I had to create something to get seniors exercising again.

That's how this book was created.

I want to motivate and educate seniors about the benefits of exercise and a healthy lifestyle. I aim to persuade people that retiring to the couch is no longer a viable option if they want to live the best life they can.

What Will You Learn from This Book?

Throughout this book, you will learn how to improve your strength, stability, and flexibility in older age.

I'll start by covering what strength training is and why it's so important for seniors. We'll learn how strength training benefits us physically and mentally in the short and long term.

Next, we'll learn about motivation and discipline. I'll cover what to do to get physically and mentally prepared for the journey ahead.

I'll cover how different lifestyle practices can aid your journey to a healthy lifestyle. In this section, I will go over nutrition, sleep, and mindset.

Once we're done with the basics, I'll move onto the exercises. I've listed a range of exercises that target multiple joints, upper body, lower body, core, and mobility. Each exercise has a detailed description, training tip, modifications, and advancements.

After covering the exercises, we'll see our 12-week progressive strength training plan. The 12-week plan can be broken into three phases. Each phase will have a different focus so we can progress with intention.

Finally, I'll end with a section on sustainability and progression of your training beyond the 12-weeks.

Disclaimer

The following guide has been designed to improve strength and flexibility; however, it should never be used as a substitute for personal medical advice. The advice from a registered professional should always take priority over the information outlined in this book. If you suspect bad health or are suffering from a medical condition, consult your doctor or physician before undergoing this program.

By participating in this program, we assume you are aware of all risk associated with the following exercises. All workouts should be performed in a safe environment under guided supervision. Every session should include an adequate warm-up and cool-down.

Part 1: The Basics of Strength Training

When we hear the phrase "strength training" many of us picture an athlete lifting heavy weights in the gym. Strength training has become linked to the young, athletic population. Contrary to popular belief, strength training can and should be performed by people of all ages.

What Is Strength Training?

Before I get into how strength training benefits seniors, let's first clarify what strength training is. Strength training represents exercises using resistance to stimulate muscular contraction, build muscle, increase strength, and improve anaerobic capacity.

Strength training uses resistance, but not specifically weights. We can use our body weight to provide resistance to an exercise. Therefore, strength training can be performed without any equipment from the comfort of our own home. However, the addition of weights can help with our progress over time. But, don't worry, you don't have to go out and buy any fancy pieces of gym equipment. You can use various items such as bottles, cans, or backpacks filled with books as weights.

Why Should Seniors Start Strength Training?

I mentioned people at any age can benefit from strength training, but it's arguably more beneficial to seniors. You might have noticed people tend to lose muscle when they age. Why? Well, in part usually due to decreased physical activity, but also because we are just predisposed to lose muscle mass and strength the older we get.

Various biological changes occur throughout our life span that lead to reductions in muscle mass, strength, and function. This represents an age-related loss of muscle mass, strength, and function, known as sarcopenia. Sarcopenia begins at just age 30 and accelerates after age 60.

You might be thinking, "Why should I care about my strength when I'm older? I'm not looking to compete in sports!". Strength is much more than sports performance and looking good. It's vital for everyday life. Take standing up out of your chair or gripping a carton of milk, for example, which requires a certain amount of strength. What might seem like an easy task now might not be possible if your strength continues to decline over time.

Think about it, the more muscle and strength we lose, the more likely our independence and quality of life will decrease. Additionally, the more susceptible we become to injury as a result of falls, etc.

Put simply, we become more fragile and are more susceptible to injury as we age. Even if you've lived a healthy life in the absence of disease, you're still suspecting the effects of aging on muscle mass and strength. Although, if you've experienced a chronic health condition such as cardiovascular disease or metabolic disease, your vulnerability becomes exacerbated.

Sarcopenia is caused by multiple mechanisms, including impaired muscle building, chronic inflammation, and disuse. Unfortunately, impaired muscle building and chronic inflammation are inevitable with aging, so we can't entirely prevent the loss of muscle mass, strength, and function. But we can limit the loss by reducing the effects of impaired muscle building and chronic inflammation. Most notably, we can prevent disuse by performing regular strength training - that's where this book can help you.

Strength training requires the use of muscles. While we can't reverse or stop the effects of aging on muscle loss, we can delay its progression, allowing us to live a more independent, high-quality life with less risk of injury.

So far, we've established that strength training is pretty good for us. It helps delay the effects of age-related muscle loss, and it also helps improve our physical and mental health. Let's have a look at how strength training affects us in the short and long term.

<u>Immediate Benefits of Strength Training</u>

During a strength training session, our bodies demand more oxygen due to an increased workload. Therefore, we begin breathing heavier to get more oxygen into the blood. The heart then needs to beat faster to deliver the oxygen to our working muscles, causing our heart rate and blood pressure to increase temporarily. Our muscles also develop micro-tears but don't worry, this is expected. To gain fitness and strength, our body has to be temporarily damaged so it can recover and come back stronger. Without this slight damage, it would not be able to adapt to a higher level of exercise.

I'm sure you can recall a time where you felt euphoric after an exercise session, right? This is due to the various endorphins we release during a workout. These endorphins make us feel happier, more energetic, and self-confident. Strength training also relieves stress by releasing tension in our bodies.

Long Term Benefits of Strength Training

Straight after a strength session, your mind feels great, but your body might feel a bit tired. Over time, we recover from this fatigue to build a higher level of fitness. We begin to build a stronger cardiopulmonary system, meaning our heart and lungs get stronger, so they don't have to work as hard at rest. Consequently, our blood pressure, breathing rate, and heart rate all decrease. Therefore, less stress is placed on our heart and lungs, meaning we're at a lower risk of developing chronic diseases, and everyday tasks feel easier.

Strength training has also been shown to:

- Reduce the effects on age-related changes in muscle mass and function loss
- Enhance muscle strength, power, and neuromuscular functioning
- Increase flexibility and mobility
- Mediate the effects of chronic inflammation

Regular exercise can improve your mental health too. It's linked to positive effects on your brain functioning and mental conditions such as stress and depression.

Part 2: Getting Started

After reading about all the benefits of strength training, I'm sure you're eager to get started. Let's get into it.

How to Start the Journey

We all know a bit of exercise is good for us, so why don't we always do it? One of the biggest reasons is poor motivation and discipline. If we're going to stick with something, we have to learn discipline and motivation.

Discipline and motivation go hand in hand. One doesn't work without the other. Motivation gives us bursts of energy but isn't always reliable on our off days. That's where discipline comes in. When we have discipline, we can get through the days when we aren't feeling motivated.

Here are some strategies you can use to add discipline and motivation into your life.

Find Your Why
First, determine why you want to make this lifestyle change, then think about that when you make a choice surrounding your health. Do you want to be fit to play with your grandkids? Or maybe you want to live an independent life? If you don't feel like performing a workout, tell yourself, "If I do this, I can become stronger and therefore won't have to rely on others to take care of me".

Set Goals
Set SMART goals. Specific, measurable, attainable, realistic, time-bound goals. SMART goals are much more effective than saying loose statements like "I want to be healthier". Instead, say I want to improve my strength and flexibility over the next 12-weeks.

Be Prepared
Exercising late in the evening isn't fun for anyone. Fit your workout into your routine. Find a time when you know

you're not going to be disturbed and can focus on the task at hand.

Build Healthy Habits
Habits are things we do regularly, often subconsciously. Implementing healthy habits into your life is an easy way to improve your health. Over time, you won't even think about doing these things. My favorite habits are drinking a glass of water every morning, going for a 10-minute walk daily, and eating vegetables with my dinner. Set yourself realistic healthy habits and try and perform them every day.

Make It Fun
A healthy lifestyle doesn't have to be boring. Make it fun by finding a workout buddy or playing your favorite music during your workout. Get creative in the kitchen and find some healthy recipes that you'll enjoy and look forward to eating.

How to Prepare Before the Exercises

Exercise is an important part of the puzzle, but a healthy lifestyle includes your sleep, nutrition, and mindset. If we don't take care of these, no amount of exercise will make up for it.

Sleep
Sleep is an essential part of our life. It lets our mind and body recover and recharge from the day's activity. A lack of sleep impairs our cognitive and physical functioning. Older adults need 7-8 hours of good quality sleep per night.

Here are a few things you can do to promote good sleeping habits:

- Set a consistent wake-up and bedtime.
- Use blackout blinds.
- Avoid your screen before bed.
- Avoid caffeine, alcohol, and large meals leading up to your bedtime.
- Sleep in a cool room.
- Make your sleeping environment peaceful and comfortable.
- Don't exercise too close to bedtime.

Nutrition
Nutrition is the foundation of a healthy lifestyle. Eating the right foods can help protect us from disease and allow us to live an optimal lifestyle. The World Health Organization (WHO) recommends we eat a diet that includes:

- Staples like cereals (wheat, barley, rye, maize or rice) or starchy tubers or roots (potato, yam, taro or cassava).
- Legumes (lentils and beans).
- Fruit and vegetables.
- Foods from animal sources (meat, fish, eggs, and milk).

Mindset

We live in our minds and bodies. But, it's often the mind we listen to the most. Therefore, our everyday mindset is a key component of a healthy lifestyle. The way we view the world we live in has a drastic effect on how we approach it, and our mind has the power to do anything.

If we want to get stronger and fitter, we change our diet and exercise regime. If we can't change our exercise regime due to injury, we can use that time to learn about rehabilitation and what we can do to come back from injury.

One way to change your mindset is to meditate. Meditation involves building a positive relationship with your thoughts. The aim is not to ignore our thoughts but rather accept and deal with them. All you need for meditation is a spare few minutes and a bit of peace. Sit in a comfortable position and start counting your breaths. Every time a thought enters your mind, recognize it, then let it pass.

Part 3: Fundamental Exercises

Throughout this book, we've included a range of exercises that can be divided into multi-joint, upper body, lower body, core, and mobility exercises. A lot of exercises will fall into more than one category, but we've placed it in its most prominent category for the purpose of this book.

Multi-Joint Exercises

Multi-joint exercises use multiple muscles or muscle groups at one time. The squat and press is a full-body exercise working the upper and lower body. Multi-joint exercises are great at replicating day-to-day tasks. For example, imagine you're lying on the floor; you will need to use all your muscles to get back on your feet.

1. Air Squats

Air squats are a multi-joint exercise working your leg muscles, including the glutes, quads, hamstrings, calves, and core. Squatting is needed for a range of everyday tasks, from standing up from your chair to picking something up off the floor.

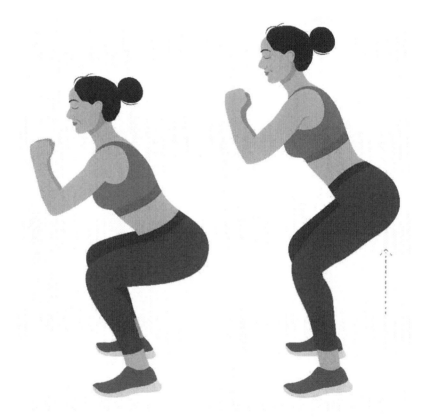

Instructions:

1. To perform the air squat, stand with your feet shoulder-width apart.
2. Push your hips back and bend the knees until your buttock is lower than your knees.

3. Keep your back straight and core engaged throughout the exercise.
4. Drive through your midfoot to return to standing.
5. During extension, push your knees out.

Tip: When setting up for the air squat, "screw" your feet into the floor.

Easier Option: Lower your buttock ¼ of the way down, rather than below your hips.

Harder Option: Add weight or add a jump during extension.

2. Squat Jumps

Squat jumps are an advanced version of air squats. Squat jumps work the hips, glutes, core, and hamstrings while improving your strength, balance, and power.

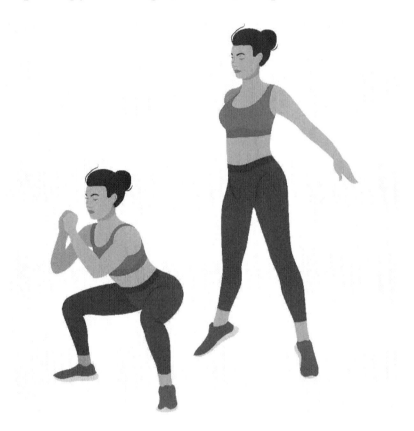

Instructions:

1. Stand with feet shoulder-width apart.
2. Send your hips back then bend at the knees until your hips are just above knee height.
3. Keep your back straight and core engaged throughout.

4. Drive through your midfoot while pushing your knees out and jump in the air.
5. When you land, slightly bend your knees upon impact to create a soft landing.

Tip: Jump as high as you comfortably can with each repetition.

Easier Option: Perform regular air squats.

Harder Option: Try rebounding your jumps. As you land, descend straight into the next repetition instead of resetting each time.

3. High Knees

High knees will ramp up your heart rate while working the glutes, quads, hamstrings, core, and calves. High knees cross over well to running, so will prepare you for when you need to run for the bus or chase your grandchildren around the garden.

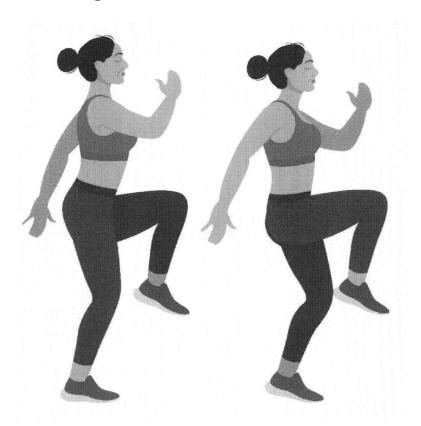

Instructions:

1. Start with your feet hip-width apart.
2. Raise your right knee up to your chest, then lower back to the floor.
3. Repeat this movement on your left leg.

4. When you get comfortable, simultaneously drive up with one leg while lowering with the other - just like you're running.

Tip: Put your hands straight out in front of your chest. Aim to hit your palms with your knee each rep.

Easier Option: Try to bring your knees up to hip height or as high as comfortable.

Harder Option: Use your arms to replicate a sprinting motion.

4. Jumping Jacks

Jumping jacks are a total-body exercise specifically focusing on your hips, lower back, thighs, shoulders, and hamstrings. They are also great for building bone strength and improving cardiovascular fitness.

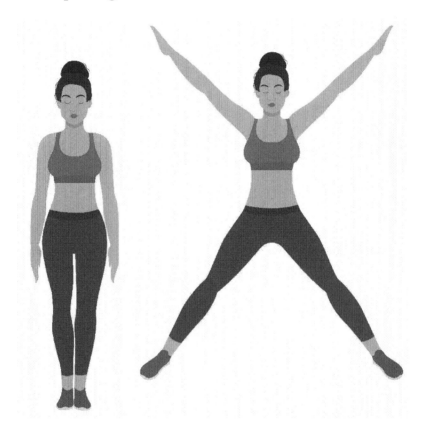

Instructions:

1. Stand with your feet shoulder-width apart, then jump into the air while moving your arms and legs away from your body.
2. You should land in a star shape with your arms and legs extended.

3. Jump back into the air while bringing your arms and legs back to the body.
4. Keep your core tight and back straight throughout the movement.

Tip: Keep your eyes facing forward to help you balance.

Easier Option: Step out to the side instead of jumping.

Harder Option: Begin each by touching your toes, then extending into the star shape.

5. Jumping Lunges

Jumping lunges are an advanced version of regular lunges. They improve your single-leg strength, balance, and power while working the hips, glutes, core, quads, and hamstrings.

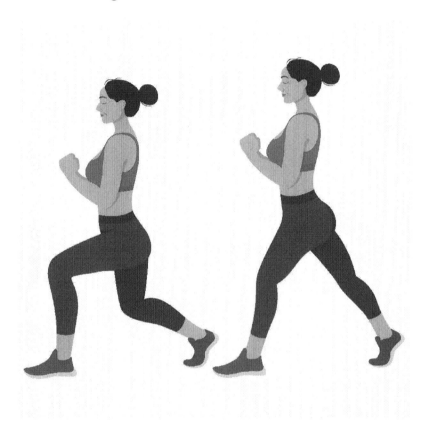

Instructions:

1. Begin standing tall with your feet hip-width apart.
2. Take a long step forward with your right foot, then lower your hips until your right knee is at a 90-degree angle.

3. Ensure your shoulders are relaxed and your core is engaged.
4. Keeping the weight in your front heel, push the floor away to jump in the air, landing in the lunge position on your left leg.
5. Alternate between legs.

Tip: Pause for a second at the bottom of the lunge to help regain your balance and stability.

Easier Option: Eliminate the jump and perform regular lunges.

Harder Option: Rebound your lunges or jump higher.

6. Mountain Climbers

Mountain climbers build your cardiovascular fitness, full-body strength, and agility. Mountain climbers place specific emphasis on the shoulders, hamstrings, quads, triceps, and core.

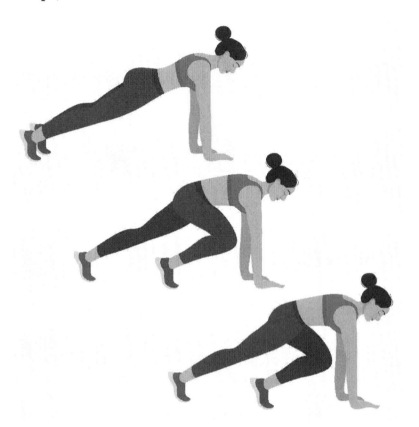

Instructions:

1. Begin in a press-up position with your arms and legs fully extended.
2. Your weight should be spread between your hands and feet.

3. Keep your shoulders, hips, and feet remain aligned throughout the movement, as well as keeping your core engaged.
4. Bring your right knee towards your right elbow.
5. Drive your right foot back to the starting position while simultaneously bringing your left knee to your chest.

Tip: Keep your neck in a neutral position. Prevent your chin from tucking in or looking to the sky.

Easier Option: Eliminate simultaneously moving your legs. Instead, bring your knee to your elbow and back again before repeating the movement on your opposite leg.

Harder Option: Instead of driving your knee to your elbow, place your foot just outside your hand. A greater range of motion will enhance your flexibility as well as strength.

7. Long Lunge

The long lunge is a quad-dominant exercise developing single-leg strength and stability. The long lunge targets your quadriceps, thighs, hips, and glutes.

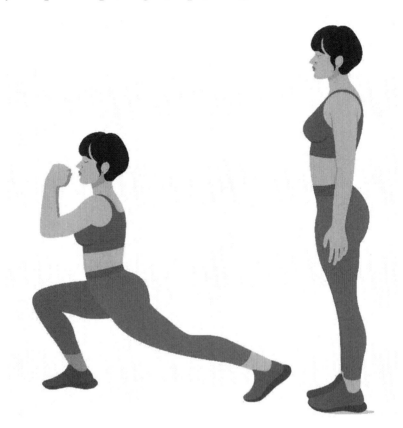

Instructions:

1. Begin standing tall with your feet shoulder-width apart.
2. Take a long step forward with your right foot while keeping your left foot planted.
3. Bend your right leg until it creates a 90-degree angle at the knee.

4. Ensure your shoulders are relaxed and your core is engaged.
5. Keeping the weight in your front heel, push the floor away to come back to your starting position.
6. Repeat the exercise on your opposite leg.

Tip: Keep your pelvis neutral, your chest high, and your back straight.

Easier Option: Feel free to cut back on the range of motion and stay above a 90-degree angle.

Harder Option: Hold weights at your side or wear a weighted backpack.

8. Kneeling Shoulder Press

The kneeling shoulder press is an excellent exercise for building upper body and core strength. Similar to a regular shoulder press, but the kneeling position provides instability which forces your core to work.

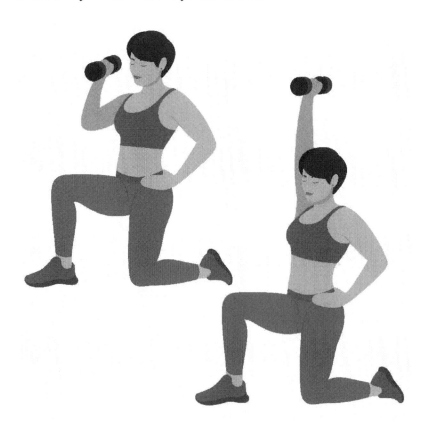

Instructions:

1. Stand tall with your feet hip-width apart and a weight in your right hand.
2. Bend your right arm to bring the weight to your shoulder.

3. Take a long step forward with your left leg, lowering the hips until your right knee touched the floor.
4. Squeeze your core and buttock tight.
5. Push the weight above your head to full extension at the elbow.
6. Pause for a second, then slowly lower back to your shoulder.
7. Repeat half the reps on your right arm before switching to your left side.

Tip: Place your opposite hand on your hip to remain balanced.

Easier Option: Perform the exercise without weights.

Harder Option: Perform the exercise with a weight in each hand.

9. Deadlift

The deadlift is one of the best exercises for building full-body strength. The deadlift primarily trains the muscles in your legs, lower back, and core. It is also a great exercise to improve your posture. During the deadlift, you need to engage your shoulders, spine, and hips. This crosses over into good posture.

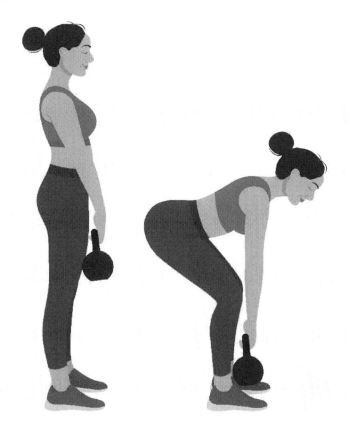

Instructions:

1. Begin standing tall with your feet hip-width apart.
2. Hold a weight in each hand at your sides.

3. Pull your shoulder blades together and engage your core.
4. Send your hips back, then bend at the knees.
5. Lower the weight as far as you can without rounding your back.
6. When you've reached maximal depth, push the hips forward to return to standing.

Tip: Keep your neck in a neutral position by looking at a spot on the floor in front of you.

Easier Option: Perform the exercise without weights.

Harder Option: Perform the deadlift with a barbell to reach greater depth.

10. Squat and Press

The squat and press is a full-body movement working the shoulders, glutes, quads, calves, hamstrings, back, and core. It is a very functional movement that has many benefits for everyday workouts.

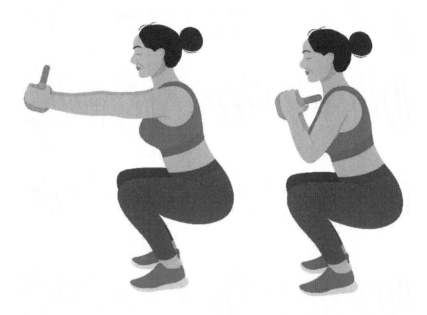

Instructions:

1. Stand tall with your feet hip-width apart with a weight held in both hands.
2. Bend the elbows to bring the weights to your shoulders; this is your starting position.

3. Pull your shoulder back, engage your core, and squeeze your buttock.
4. Push your hips back and bend the knees until your buttock is lower than your knees.
5. Keep your back straight and core engaged throughout the exercise.
6. At the bottom of the squat, push your weight out until your arms reach full extension.
7. Pause for one second before bringing the weight back to your chest.
8. Drive through your midfoot to return to standing.
9. During extension, push your knees out.

Tip: To make things appear more manageable, focus on performing the squat and press as individual exercises.

Easier Option: Perform the exercise without the weight.

Harder Option: Keep the weight extended out for the duration of the squat.

11. Lunge and Press

The lunge and press is a full-body movement working the shoulders, chest, glutes, quads, calves, hamstrings, back, and core. The main benefit of the lunge and press is single-limb strength development. It's important to keep your strength balanced to reduce the risk of injury.

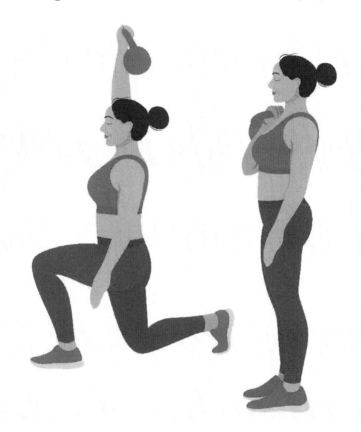

Instructions:

1. Stand tall with your feet hip-width apart with a weight in your left hand.
2. Bend the elbow to bring the weights to your shoulder; this is your starting position.

3. Pull your shoulder back, engage your core, and squeeze your buttock.
4. Take a long step forward with your right foot while keeping your left foot planted.
5. Bend your right leg until it creates a 90-degree angle at the knee.
6. While bending your leg, push the weight towards the sky until your arm reaches full extension.
7. Keeping the weight in your front heel, push through the floor and lower the weight to come back to your starting position.
8. Perform half the repetitions on one side and the remaining on the opposite side.

Tip: Hold your non-working arm out to the side to aid balance.

Easier Option: Perform the exercise without the weight.

Harder Option: Perform the exercise with a weight in both hands.

12. Plank Hops

Plank hops strengthen your core and cardiovascular system. They also help build strength in the shoulders, glutes, quads, hamstrings, and triceps.

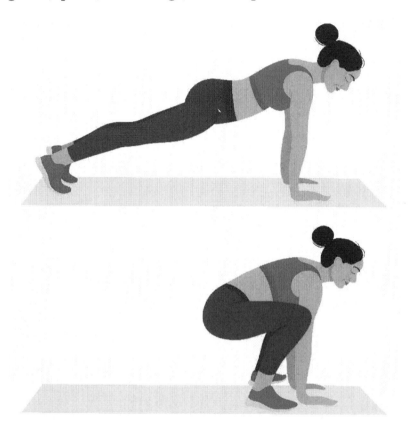

Instructions:

1. Start in the plank position.
2. Place your hands under your shoulders and toes on the floor.
3. Your shoulders, buttock, and ankles should all be aligned.
4. Squeeze your core and buttock.

5. Jump your feet to land below your buttock.
6. Briefly pause before jumping back to the plank position.

Tip: Keep your feet together.

Easier Option: Step each leg in rather than jump.

Harder Option: Rebound the jumps without pausing between them.

13. Plank Jacks

Plank jacks improve full-body stability and strengthen your cardiovascular system, spine, back, core, glutes, hamstrings, shoulders, abductors, adductors, and triceps.

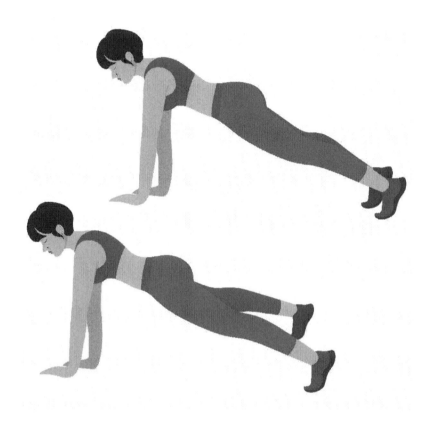

Instructions:

1. Start in the plank position.
2. Place your hands under your shoulders and toes on the floor.
3. Your shoulders, buttock, and ankles should all be aligned.
4. Squeeze your core and buttock.

5. Jump your feet out wide, pause for a second, then jump back to the center.

Tip: Imagine you're performing a jumping jack in the plank position.

Easier Option: Step your feet out wide instead of jumping.

Harder Option: Rebound your jumps by not pausing.

14. Weight Hold and Squat

The weight hold and squat is a full-body movement working the shoulders, glutes, quads, calves, hamstrings, back, and core. Keeping the weight held out puts more emphasis on your shoulder muscles.

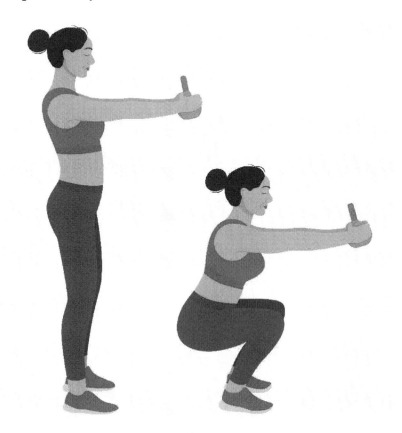

Instructions:

1. Stand tall with your feet hip-width apart with a weight held in both hands.
2. Push your weight out until your arms reach full extension - this is your starting position.

3. Pull your shoulder back, engage your core, and squeeze your buttock.
4. Push your hips back and bend the knees until your buttock is lower than your knees.
5. Keep your back straight and core engaged throughout the exercise.
6. Drive through your midfoot to return to standing.
7. During extension, push your knees out.

Tip: Keep your eyes on your weight to help with balance.

Easier Option: Perform the exercise without the weight.

Harder Option: Pause at the bottom of the squat for two seconds.

15. Burpees

Burpees are a full-body exercise working your core, shoulders, legs, and back. They are also a great movement for strengthening your cardiovascular system.

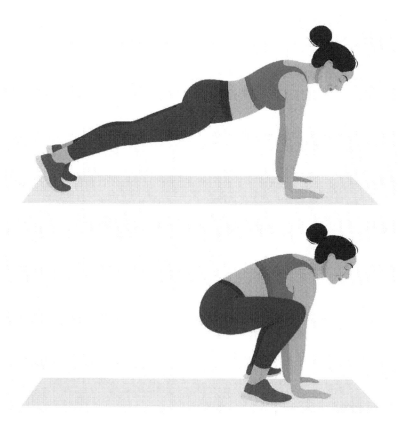

Instructions:

1. Stand tall with your feet shoulder-width apart.
2. Squeeze your core and buttock.
3. Send your hips back and lower your hands to the floor.
4. Jump your feet back to a plank position.

5. Your shoulders, buttock, and ankles should all be aligned.
6. Briefly pause, then jump your feet to the land below your buttock.
7. Extend your hips and jump to full extension.

Tip: Ensure your weight is over your shoulders before jumping back.

Easier Option: Step your feet back rather than jump.

Harder Option: Perform a press-up when in the plank position.

16. Single Leg Box Squat

Single leg box squats are similar to bench squats but focus on single-limb movement. Single limb movements help eliminate any muscle imbalances. The single leg box squat develops strength in your glutes, hamstrings, and quads. This is a great crossover to real-life movements such as standing up out of a chair. If you don't have a box, use a raised surface of similar height, such as a chair, bench, or low wall.

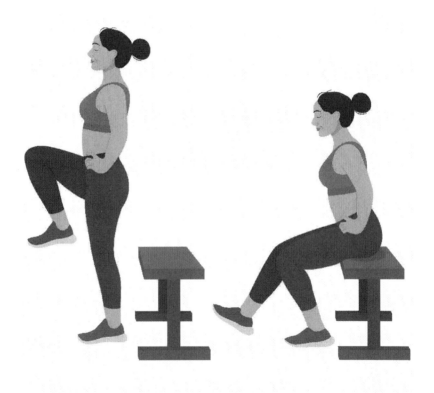

Instructions:

1. To perform the single leg box squat, stand with feet shoulder-width apart.
2. Squeeze your shoulder blades, core, and buttock.
3. Lift your right leg off the floor an inch or two.
4. Send your hips back and bend your left knee until you are sitting on the bench.
5. After a brief pause, drive your hips up to return to standing while keeping your core tight and back neutral.
6. Perform half the repetitions on your left leg and half on your right.

Tip: It's important to pause on the box. This exercise aims to eliminate any rebound movement.

Easier Option: Perform regular bench squats.

Harder Option: Hold a weight at chest height.

17. Single Leg Raise

Single leg raises are an advanced version of plank hip dips. They develop full-body strength and stability. The additional hip raise also puts more emphasis on the glutes.

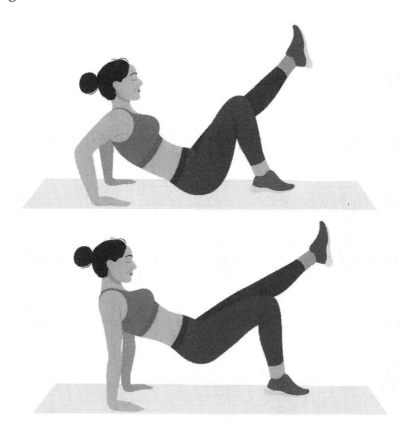

Instructions:

1. Begin sitting on the floor with your legs extended and torso upright.
2. Place your hands on the floor behind your shoulders.

3. Lean back so your arms take the weight of your body.
4. Bring your feet to your buttock while remaining flat on the floor.
5. Push through your feet and palms to lift your hips slightly off the floor.
6. From here, fully extend your left leg towards the sky.
7. Lift your hip and extend your arms.
8. Pause for one second, then lower back to the floor.
9. Perform half the repetitions on your right leg and half on your left.

Tip: Push through your foot on the floor to assist the lift.

Easier Option: Keep both feet on the floor.

Harder Option: Place a resistance band just above your knees.

18. Knee to Elbow Extension

Knee to elbow extensions are similar to mountain climbers but focus more on the glutes. They also work your shoulders, hamstrings, quads, triceps, and core.

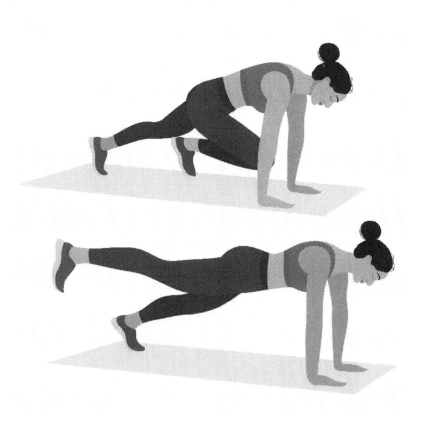

Instructions:

1. Begin in a press up position with your arms and legs fully extended.
2. Your weight should be spread between your hands and feet.

3. Keep your shoulders, hips, and feet remain aligned throughout the movement, as well as keeping your core engaged.
4. Bring your right knee towards your right elbow.
5. Drive your right foot back and raise your foot to the sky.
6. Pause for a second before returning to the starting position.
7. Repeat the movement on your left leg.

Tip: Lift your leg until you feel your glute fully contract.

Easier Option: Only perform the leg lift, do not bring your knee to your elbow.

Harder Option: Place a resistance band just above your knees.

19. Lunge Jumps

Lunge jumps are a core, glute, hip flexor, and hamstring focused exercise. They're similar to reverse lunges but have an additional single-leg jump.

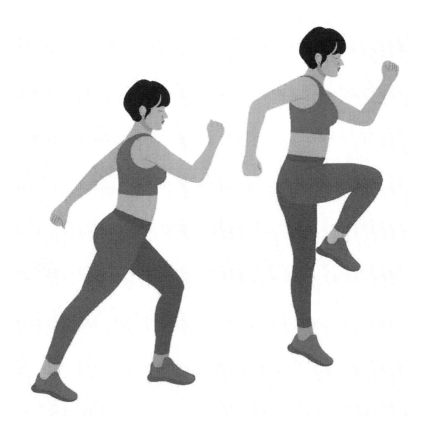

Instructions:

1. Begin standing with your feet hip-width apart.
2. Take a long step back with your right leg and bend your left knee until it reaches a 90-degree angle.
3. Keep your core and buttocks tight.
4. Drive through the midfoot of your left leg to return to standing.

5. In the same motion, bring your right knee to your chest while performing a small jump on your left leg.
6. Return to the starting position before repeating on the opposite side.

Tip: Focus on a specific place on the wall throughout the exercise to help with your balance.

Easier Option: Eliminate the jump.

Harder Option: Hold a weight in each hand.

20. Swimmers

Swimmers are an advanced version of alternating superman. They work single limb strength and stability in your upper back, lower back, glutes, hamstrings, and core. It's a great exercise for improving posture and alleviating back pain.

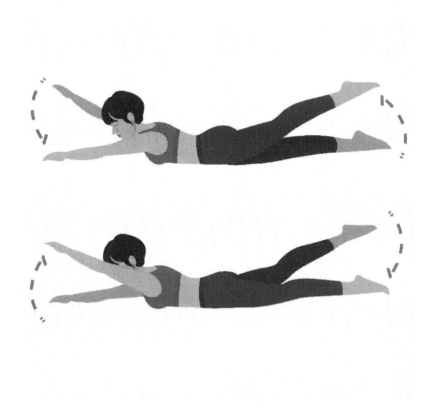

Instructions:

1. Begin lying face down with your legs extended and arms above your head.
2. Push your hips into the floor while squeezing your core and buttocks.

3. Lift your arms and feet off the floor slightly - this is your starting position.
4. Lift your right arm and left foot as far as you comfortably can.
5. Lower to the starting position while simultaneously lifting your left arm and right foot.

Tip: Think of the action like a front crawl.

Easier Option: Perform alternating superman.

Harder Option: Hold a weight in each hand.

Upper Body Exercises

Upper body exercises build strength in the shoulders, biceps, triceps, chest, and back. They are helpful for everyday activities such as reaching, pulling, pushing, and lifting.

21. Tricep Dips

Tricep dips are an upper body exercise focusing on the backs of your arms. Our triceps help us extend our arms.

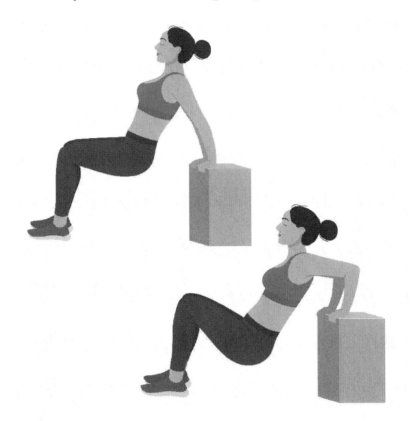

Instructions:

1. To perform a tricep dip, you'll need a raised surface such as a chair or a bench.
2. Edge your buttock just off the side of the surface, so your feet are flat on the floor.
3. Bend your elbows until they form a 90-degree angle, then push through your palm to return to extension.

Tip: Look forward rather than down at your feet to keep your neck in a neutral position.

Easier Option: Bring your feet closer to the elevated surface.

Harder Option: Move your feet further from the elevated surface.

22. Bicep Curl

Bicep curls build pulling strength in the arms. They also help build strength in your forearms which crosses over into a stronger grip. A strong grip is needed in everyday tasks such as opening jars.

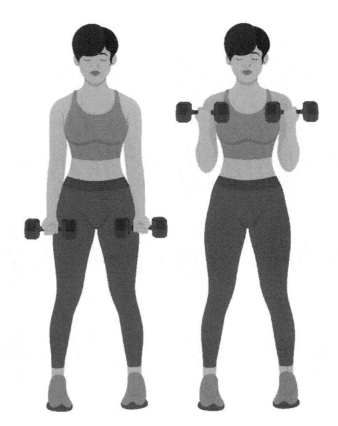

Instructions:

1. Stand tall with your feet hip-width apart.
2. Hold a weight in each hand with your arms fully extended at your side.
3. Embrace your core and buttock.

4. Rotate your hands in so your palms are facing forwards.
5. Bend at the elbow to bring the weight up to your shoulder.
6. Hold for a second before slowly lowering the weight back down.
7. Ensure your elbows remain pinned to your side.

Tip: Do not swing the weight to generate momentum; this takes the tension out of the exercise and makes it less effective.

Easier Option: Perform the exercise without weights.

Harder Option: Lower the weight for a count of three seconds.

23. Hammer Curl

The hammer curl is a variation of the traditional bicep curl. However, your wrist remains in a fixed position to target additional muscles in your upper and lower arms.

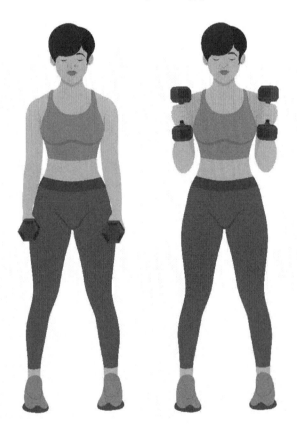

Instructions:

1. Stand tall with your feet hip-width apart.
2. Hold a weight in each hand with your arms fully extended at your side.
3. Embrace your core and buttock.
4. Keep your palms facing your body and wrists held tight.

5. Bend at the elbow to bring the weight up to your shoulder.
6. Hold for a second before slowly lowering the weight back down.
7. Ensure your elbows remain pinned to your side.

Tip: Keep your wrists tight to work the smaller muscles in your hands. Don't let your wrists flop.

Easier Option: Perform the exercise without weights.

Harder Option: Lower the weight for a count of three seconds.

24. Shoulder Press

The shoulder press strengthens your shoulders and upper back. It's an excellent crossover for overhead press movement, such as putting your bag into overhead storage.

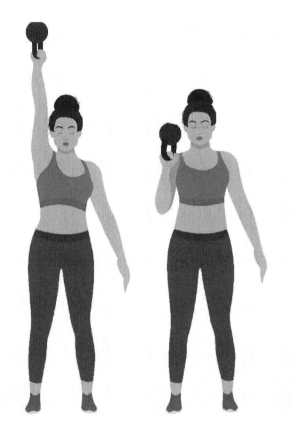

Instructions:

1. Stand tall with your feet hip-width apart with a weight in each hand.
2. Bend the elbows to bring the weights to your shoulders; this is your starting position.

3. Pull your shoulder back, engage your core, and squeeze your buttock.
4. Push the weights towards the sky until they reach full extension.
5. Pause for one second, then lower the weights back to the starting position.

Tip: Push your head forward during extension.

Easier Option: Perform the exercise without weights.

Harder Option: Perform the exercise on the floor with your legs extended and torso upright.

<u>25. Front Raises</u>

Front raises focus on building your shoulder strength, specifically your anterior shoulder strength. They also help strengthen the shoulder joint.

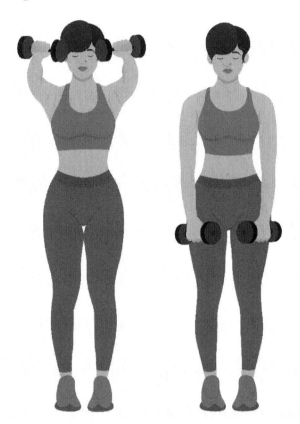

Instructions:

1. Stand tall with your feet hip-width apart and a weight in each hand at your sides.
2. Pull your shoulders back, squeeze your buttock, and engage your core.

3. Slightly bend your elbows, then lift the weight out in front of you until your arms are parallel to the floor.
4. Pause for one second, then slowly lower back to the center.

Tip: Keep your wrists tight, don't let them get sloppy.

Easier Option: Perform the exercise without the weights.

Harder Option: Slow down the movement by counting to three during the lowering phase.

26. Lateral Raises

Lateral raises focus on building your shoulder strength, specifically your lateral shoulder strength. They also help strengthen the shoulder joint.

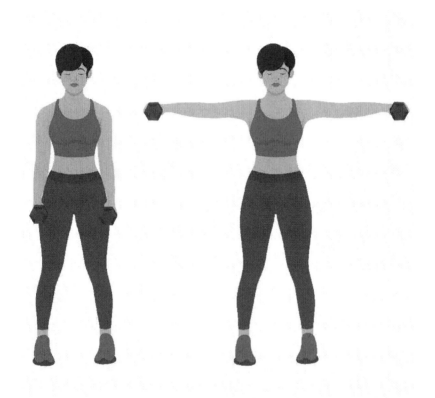

Instructions:

1. Stand tall with your feet hip-width apart and a weight in each hand at your sides.
2. Pull your shoulders back, squeeze your buttock, and engage your core.
3. Slightly bend your elbows, then lift the weight out to the side until your arms are parallel to the floor.

76

4. Pause for one second, then slowly lower back to the center.

Tip: Initiate the movement with your elbows.

Easier Option: Perform the exercise without the weights.

Harder Option: Reduce the range of motion to keep tension in the shoulders.

27. Single Arm Lateral Raises

Similar to regular lateral raises, single-arm lateral raises focus on building your shoulder strength, specifically your lateral shoulder strength. They also help strengthen the shoulder joint. However, performing one arm at a time works your core more.

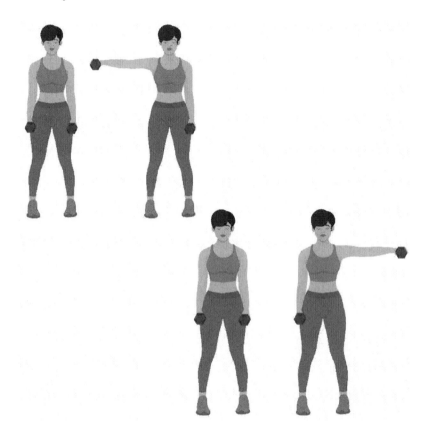

Instructions:

1. Stand tall with your feet hip-width apart and a weight in your right hand at your side.
2. Pull your shoulders back, squeeze your buttock, and engage your core.

3. Slightly bend your elbows, then lift your right arm out to the side until your arm is parallel to the floor.
4. Pause for one second, then slowly lower back to the center.
5. Repeat the movement on your left arm.
6. Continue alternating between your right and left arm.

Tip: Keep your torso straight, fight the urge to bend from side to side.

Easier Option: Perform the exercise without the weights.

Harder Option: Stand pressed against a wall to isolate your shoulder muscle further.

28. Front to Lateral Raises

Front to lateral raises reaps the benefits of both exercises. It develops your single-arm shoulder strength, specifically your lateral and anterior shoulder strength. They also help strengthen the shoulder joint.

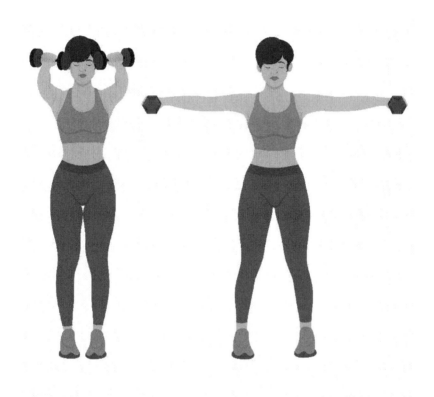

Instructions:

1. Stand tall with your feet hip-width apart and a weight in each hand at your sides.
2. Pull your shoulders back, squeeze your buttock, and engage your core.

3. Slightly bend your elbows, then lift the weight out in front of you until your arms are parallel to the floor.
4. Pause for one second, then slowly lower back to the center.
5. Then, lift the weight out to the side until your arms are parallel to the floor.
6. Pause for one second, then slowly lower back to the center. Continue alternating between front and lateral raises.

Tip: Imagine your hips are fixed in one position. Don't let them swing forward to create momentum.

Easier Option: Perform the exercise without the weights.

Harder Option: Perform two lateral raises for every one front raise.

29. Plank Raises

The plank improves full-body stability and strengthens your spine, back, core, glutes, hamstrings, shoulders, and triceps. The plank raises places particular emphasis on developing shoulder strength.

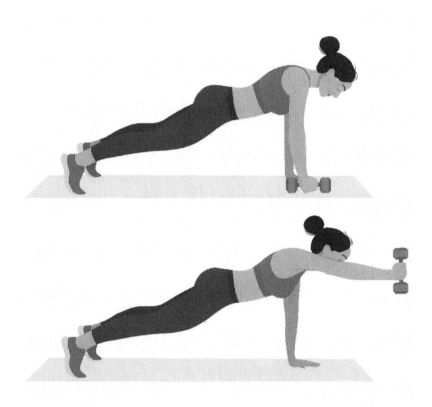

Instructions:

1. Start in the plank position with a weight next to each hand.
2. Place your hands under your shoulders and toes on the floor.

3. Your shoulders, buttock, and ankles should all be aligned.
4. Squeeze your core and buttock.
5. Shift your weight onto your left side while gripping the weight in your right hand.
6. Keeping your arm extended, raise the weight until it is parallel to the floor.
7. Briefly pause before lowering back to the starting position.
8. Repeat the movement on your opposite side.

Tip: Slowly shift your weight to one side to maintain balance.

Easier Option: Perform the exercise on your knees without weights.

Harder Option: Do not alternate. Perform half the repetitions on one side before completing the other half on the opposite side.

30. Plank Toe Taps

The plank improves full-body stability and strengthens your spine, back, core, glutes, hamstrings, shoulders, and triceps. Plank toe taps place greater emphasis on the abdominals and obliques and help improve hip mobility.

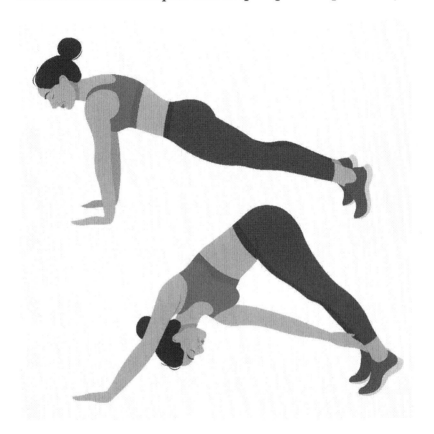

Instructions:

1. Start in the plank position.
2. Place your hands under your shoulders and toes on the floor.
3. Your shoulders, buttock, and ankles should all be aligned.

4. Squeeze your core and buttock.
5. Lift your hips towards the sky and touch your left foot with your right hand.
6. Your feet and left hand should stay in place.
7. Slowly lower your hips back to the starting position before repeating the exercise on the opposite side.
8. Continue alternating.

Tip: Be careful not to drop your hips too low during the descent.

Easier Option: Move your hands as close to your toes as possible.

Harder Option: Do not alternate. Perform half the repetitions on one side before completing the other half on the opposite side.

31. Bird Dog Plank

The bird dog plank improves full-body stability and strengthens your spine, back, core, glutes, hamstrings, shoulders, and triceps. Transferring your weight onto single limbs is a great way to build joint strength and control.

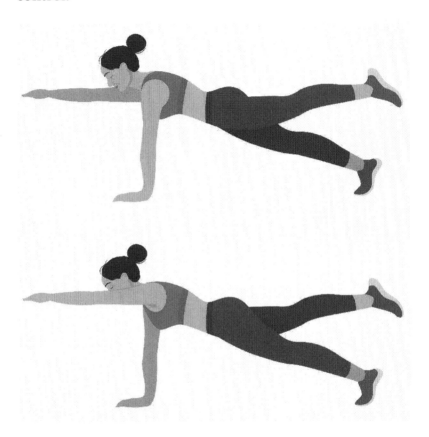

Instructions:

1. Start in the plank position.
2. Place your hands under your shoulders and toes on the floor.

3. Your shoulders, buttock, and ankles should all be aligned.
4. Squeeze your core and buttock.
5. Extend your right leg and left arm until they are parallel to the floor.
6. Hold for two seconds before returning to the starting position.
7. Repeat on the opposite side.

Tip: Practice shifting your weight onto your arms before getting your legs involved.

Easier Option: Raise your legs only.

Harder Option: Hold for five seconds at the top of the movement.

32. Plank Row

The plank row is a full-body strength-building exercise. The plank row targets the mid and upper back, shoulders, arms, and core.

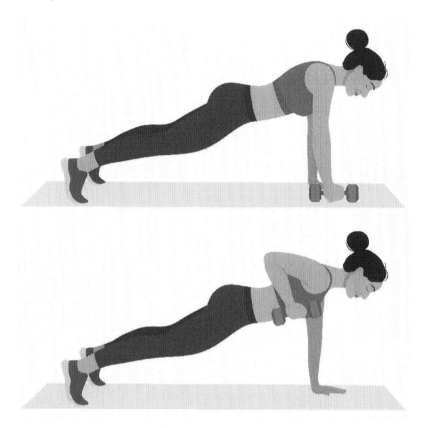

Instructions:

1. Start in the plank position with a weight next to each hand.
2. Place your hands under your shoulders and toes on the floor.
3. Your shoulders, buttock, and ankles should all be aligned.

4. Squeeze your core and buttock.
5. Shift your weight onto your left side while gripping the weight in your right hand.
6. Pull the weight up to your chest and hold for two seconds before slowly lowering it.
7. Perform half the repetitions on your right arm before completing half on the left.

Tip: Imagine you are pulling your shoulder blade to the center of your back.

Easier Option: Perform the exercise without weights.

Harder Option: Pause for four seconds at the top of the row.

33. Plank Tricep Kickbacks

The plank improves full-body stability and strengthens your spine, back, core, glutes, hamstrings, shoulders, and triceps. Plank tricep kickbacks add additional tricep resistance training to supplement pushing strength.

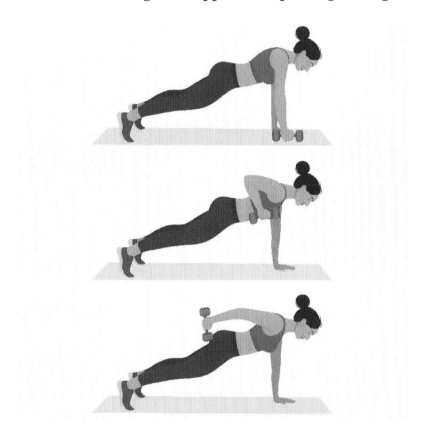

Instructions:

1. Start in the plank position with a weight next to each hand.
2. Place your hands under your shoulders and toes on the floor.

3. Your shoulders, buttock, and ankles should all be aligned.
4. Squeeze your core and buttock.
5. Shift your weight onto your left side while gripping the weight in your right hand.
6. Pull the weight up to your chest and hold.
7. Extend your arm back until the weight touches your buttock.
8. Perform half the repetitions on your right arm before completing half on the left.

Tip: Imagine your elbow is being pulled to the sky.

Easier Option: Perform the exercise on your knees without weights.

Harder Option: Keep your elbow at your side for all the repetitions instead of lowering it between.

34. Inverted Push Up

The inverted push up is an advanced version of a regular push up. It builds upper body strength and shoulder stabilization. Unlike the standard push up, the inverted push up places more emphasis on the shoulders and upper back.

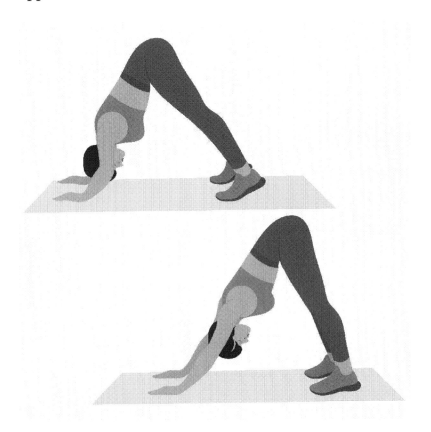

Instructions:

1. Start in the plank position.
2. Place your hands under your shoulders and toes on the floor.

3. Your shoulders, buttock, and ankles should all be aligned.
4. Squeeze your core and buttock.
5. Push your hips back into an upside-down v position.
6. Bend your elbows to lower your head to the floor.
7. Pause briefly before driving through your palms back to the starting position.

Tip: Keep your elbows pulled into the body; they should not be flaring out.

Easier Option: Perform a regular push up.

Harder Option: Bring your hands and feet closer together.

35. Press Up

The press up is one of the best bodyweight exercises for building upper body pushing strength. It helps build strength in the chest, shoulders, triceps, biceps, and back. It also helps strengthen the shoulder joint.

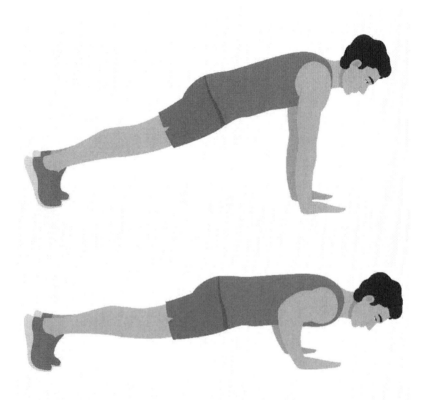

Instructions:

1. Start in the plank position.
2. Place your hands under your shoulders and toes on the floor.
3. Your shoulders, buttock, and ankles should all be aligned.

4. Squeeze your core and buttock.
5. Bend the elbows to lower your chest to the floor.
6. Pause for one second before pushing through the palms to return to the starting position.

Tip: Your hips and shoulders should move together. Don't bend your back to make the movement easier.

Easier Option: Perform the press ups on your knees.

Harder Option: Pause for four seconds at the bottom of the push up.

36. Press Up Hold

The press up hold works the same muscles as the regular press up but focuses on isometric strength (exerting force without moving the muscle). We use isometric strength when we're holding something; thus is great for everyday life.

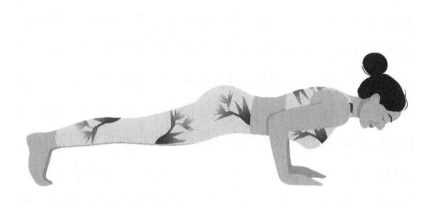

Instructions:

1. Start in the plank position.
2. Place your hands under your shoulders and toes on the floor.

3. Your shoulders, buttock, and ankles should all be aligned.
4. Squeeze your core and buttock.
5. Bend the elbows to lower your chest to the floor.
6. Hold this position.

Tip: Keep your elbows tucked into your sides, don't let them flare out.

Easier Option: Reduce the range of motion by holding further from the floor.

Harder Option: Lift one foot off the floor to test your core strength and balance.

37. Single Arm Row

The single arm row builds pulling strength in your shoulders, upper back, and core. Everyday tasks rely on pulling actions, such as opening a cupboard or door.

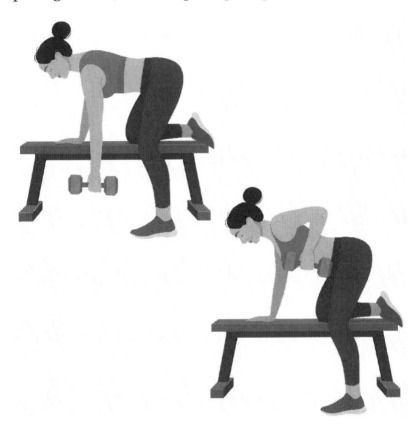

Instructions:

1. Hold a weight in your right hand.
2. Place your left hand and left knee on the side of a bench.
3. Your knee should be directly under your hips and your hand under your shoulder.

4. Draw the shoulder blades back while squeezing the glutes and core.
5. Keeping your back straight, bend your right elbow to bring the weight to your chest.
6. Pause for one second before slowly returning to extension.
7. Perform half the repetitions on your right side and half on the left.

Tip: Do not rotate the torso. Ensure all movement comes from the arm.

Easier Option: Perform the exercise without weight.

Harder Option: Pause for three seconds at the top of the movement.

38. Shrugs

Shrugs build strength in your shoulders, neck, and upper back. They also help reduce neck and shoulder strain, as well as improve posture.

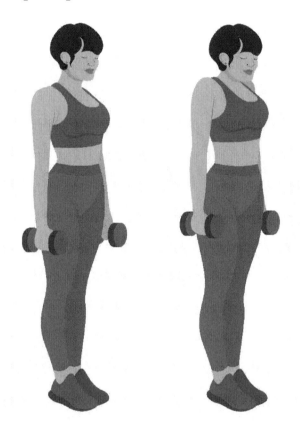

Instructions:

1. Stand tall with your feet hip-width apart.
2. Hold a weight in each hand at your sides.
3. Rotate your palms into your body.
4. Squeeze your core and buttock and draw your shoulder blades back.

5. Keeping your arms straight, lift your shoulders as high as possible.
6. Pause for one second before lowering to the starting position.

Tip: Imagine you are trying to touch your ears with your shoulders.

Easier Option: Perform the exercise without weights.

Harder Option: Perform the exercise with a barbell.

39. Split Stance Row

The split stance position improves your core and leg stability and strength. The rowing portion of the exercise works your shoulders, back, biceps, and triceps.

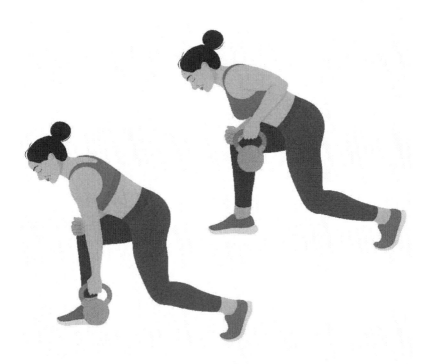

Instructions:

1. Stand tall with your feet shoulder-width apart and a weight in your right hand.
2. Step your left leg in front of you and your right leg behind - this is your split stance position.
3. Bend your left knee slightly, then lean your torso until it's close to parallel to the floor.

4. Engage your core and buttocks.
5. Bend your right elbow to pull the weight to your chest.
6. Pause for one second, then slowly lower to full extension.
7. Perform half the repetitions on your right side and the other half on your left.

Tip: Place your left hand on your left thigh for stability.

Easier Option: Perform the exercise without weights.

Harder Option: Pause for four seconds at the top of the movement.

40. Curl to External Rotation

The curl to external rotation helps build strength and stability in your biceps, shoulders, and rotator cuffs. It's important to keep our rotator cuffs strong as they're the muscles involved in shoulder joint stabilization.

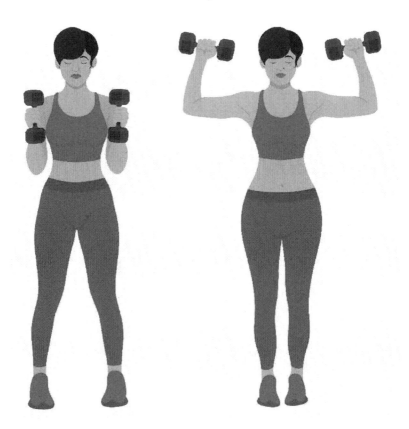

Instructions:

1. Stand tall with your feet hip-width apart.
2. Hold a weight in each hand with your arms fully extended at your side.
3. Embrace your core and buttock.

4. Rotate your hands in so your palms are facing forwards.
5. Bend at the elbow to bring the weight up to your shoulder.
6. Briefly pause.
7. From here, move your elbows out to the side until they are parallel to the floor.
8. Briefly pause.
9. Then, rotate your shoulder, so your hands are aligned with your head.
10. Briefly pause before reversing the sequence back to the starting position.

Tip: Break the movement down into three phases to make it easier to follow.

Easier Option: Perform the exercise without weights.

Harder Option: Lower the weight for a count of five seconds.

Lower Body Exercises

Lower body exercises build strength in the quads, glutes, hamstrings, and calves. They are helpful for everyday activities such as kicking, walking, pushing, and lifting.

41. Reverse Lunges

Reverse lunges are a core, glute, and hamstring focused exercise. Unlike regular lunges, we will be stepping back with our legs to initiate the movement rather than stepping forward. This places less stress on your joints and gives you more stability in your front leg. Therefore, it's a great exercise for those with knee problems, balance issues, or restricted hip mobility.

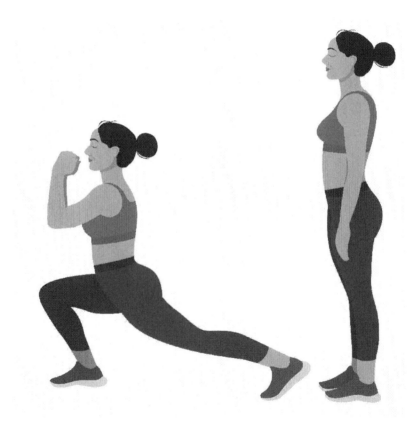

Instructions:

1. Begin standing with your feet hip-width apart.

2. Take a long step back with your right leg and bend your left knee until it reaches a 90-degree angle.
3. Keep your core and buttocks tight.
4. Drive through the midfoot of your left leg to return to standing.
5. During the drive-up, push your left knee out to the side.
6. Repeat on the opposite side.

Tip: Focus on a specific place on the wall throughout the exercise to help with your balance.

Easier Option: Reduce the range of motion by staying above a 90-degree angle.

Harder Option: Hold a weight in each hand.

42. Bulgarian Split Squats

The Bulgarian split squat is a single-leg movement working the glutes, hamstrings, hips, and quads. Single-leg movements are a great way to ensure both sides of the body have equal amounts of strength, thus helping reduce the risk of injury. During the Bulgarian split squat, your back foot is raised. Therefore, you're forced to work in a greater range of motion, allowing more focus to be placed on your quads.

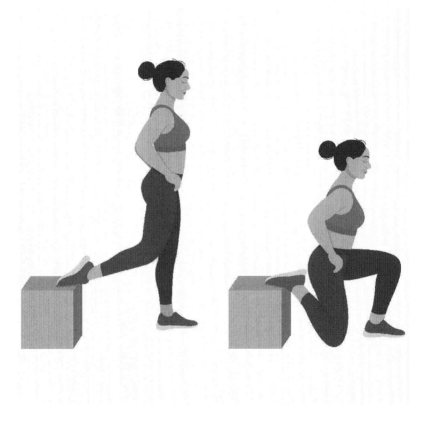

Instructions:

1. Stand with your feet shoulder-width apart.

2. Hold a weight in each hand and hold them at your side.
3. Step forward with your right leg and place your left foot on a bench behind you.
4. The top of your foot should be touching the top of the bench, allowing your ankle to flex without getting caught on the bench easily.
5. You are now in the starting position.
6. Lower your left knee to the floor while creating a 90-degree angle in your right leg.
7. Pause for 2 seconds before driving through your right midfoot to return to the starting position.
8. Repeat on your opposite side.

Tip: Tilt your torso forward slightly.

Easier Option: Perform the exercise without weights.

Harder Option: Drive through your midfoot with more power to push your foot off the floor.

43. Wide Squat

Wide squats require more hip extension than regular air squats. Thus, it places more emphasis on hip strength. However, just like normal air squats, wide squats work your glutes, quads, hamstrings, calves, and core.

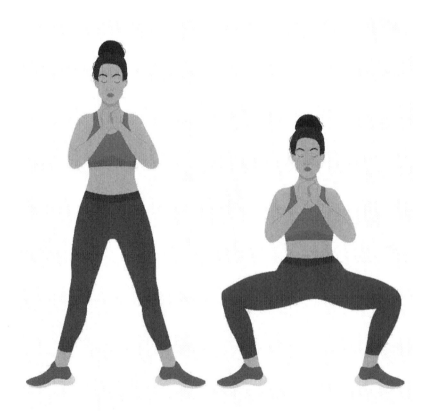

Instructions:

1. To perform the wide squat, stand with your feet outside shoulder-width apart.
2. Push your hips back and bend the knees until your buttock is just above knee height.

3. Keep your back straight and core engaged throughout the exercise.
4. Drive through your midfoot to return to standing.
5. During extension, push your knees out.

Tip: Initiate the movement from your hips, not your knees.

Easier Option: Bring your feet closer together to perform a regular air squat.

Harder Option: Hold a weight at chest height, or wear a weighted backpack.

<u>44. Bench Squats</u>

Bench squats are similar to regular squats but eliminate the use of momentum to stand back up. This is a great crossover to real-life movements such as standing up out of a chair. The bench squat develops strength in your glutes, hamstrings, and quads. If you don't have a bench, use a raised surface of similar height, such as a chair or low wall.

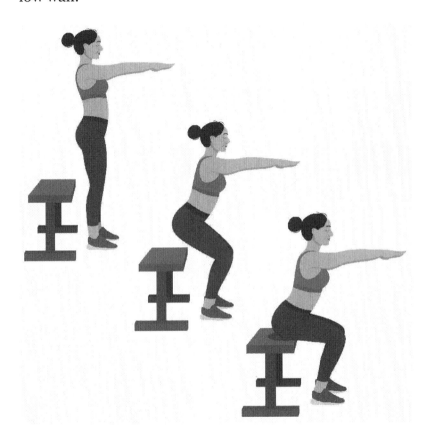

Instructions:

1. To perform the bench squat, stand with feet shoulder-width apart.

2. Squeeze your shoulder blades, core, and buttock.
3. Send your hips back and bend your knees until you are sitting on the bench.
4. After a brief pause, drive your hips up to return to standing while keeping your core tight and back neutral.

Tip: It's important to pause on the bench. This exercise aims to eliminate any rebound movement.

Easier Option: Use your hands to assist you up off the bench.

Harder Option: Hold a weight at chest height.

45. Calf Raises

Calf raises build strength in the lower legs. Lower leg strength is vital for protecting your ankles from injury.

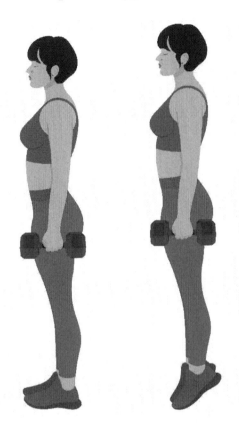

Instructions:

1. Stand tall with your feet just inside shoulder-width.
2. Point your toes forward.
3. Hold a weight in each hand.
4. Squeeze your shoulder blades together.
5. Push through the balls of the feet, raising your heels above your toes.

6. Hold for two seconds before slowly lowering.
7. Repeat this movement.

Tip: Place your toes on an elevated surface such as a book to increase the range of motion.

Easier Option: Perform the exercise without weights.

Harder Option: Do not let your feet touch the floor between reps. Keep tension in your lower leg by pausing half an inch from the floor.

46. Single Leg Deadlift

Single leg deadlifts work single leg, core, and shoulder strength. They also develop single leg balance, strength, stabilization, mobility, and posture.

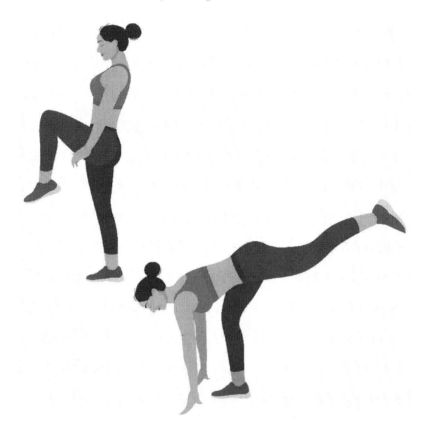

Instructions:

1. Stand tall with your feet hip-width apart.
2. Keep your hands extended at your side.
3. Pull your shoulder blades together and engage your core and buttock.
4. Slightly bend at the knees and raise your left foot off the floor, keeping your knees aligned.

5. From here, send the hips back without bending the knees. Keep your back flat, chest raised, and leg extended.
6. Lower your hand towards your toes as far as you can without rounding your back.
7. When you've reached maximal depth, push the hips forward to return to standing.
8. Repeat half the reps on one leg, then half on the opposite leg.

Tip: Pause between repetitions to regain your balance.

Easier Option: Keep both legs on the floor and perform the movement.

Harder Option: Don't let your left foot touch the floor between repetitions.

47. Weighted Single Leg Deadlift

Like regular single leg deadlifts, weighted single leg deadlifts work single leg, core, and shoulder strength. They also develop single leg balance, strength, stabilization, mobility, and posture. However, weighted single-leg deadlifts add a greater range of motion and resistance to make the exercise more challenging.

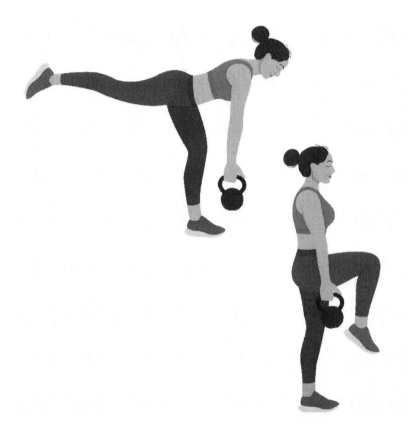

Instructions:

1. Stand tall with your feet hip-width apart.
2. Hold the weight in your left hand at your side.

3. Pull your shoulder blades together and engage your core and buttock.
4. Slightly bend at the knees and raise your left foot off the floor, keeping your knees aligned.
5. From here, send the hips back without bending the knees.
6. Keep your back flat, chest raised, and leg extended.
7. Lower your weight towards your toes as far as you can without rounding your back.
8. When you've reached maximal depth, push the hips forward to return to standing.
9. Repeat half the reps on one leg, then half on the opposite leg.

Tip: Drive through your heel during extension.

Easier Option: Perform the exercise without weight.

Harder Option: Slow the lowering phase of the exercise by counting to three.

48. Glute Bridge

The glute bridge works the glutes, core, lower back, hamstrings, and hips. The glute bridge can also be used to alleviate knee and lower back pain.

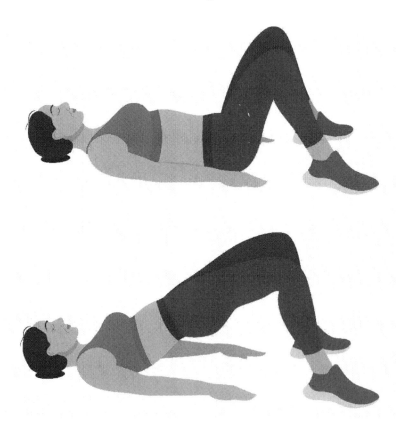

Instructions:

1. Begin lying on the floor with your legs extended and arms at your side.
2. Pull your feet to your buttock until they are flat on the floor.
3. Push your shoulders, upper back, and lower back into the floor while squeezing your core.

4. Engage your glutes, then push your hips towards the sky.
5. At the top of the movement, your knees, hips, and shoulders should be aligned.
6. Pause at the top for two seconds before slowly lowering.

Tip: Push your knees out during extension.

Easier Option: Place your feet further from your core.

Harder Option: Place a weight on your groin area.

49. Side Lunges

Side lunges help improve your balance, strength, and stability. They work your inner and outer thighs, also known as your adductors and abductors. The sideways movement helps prepare your body for side-to-side movements such as shuffling during sports play.

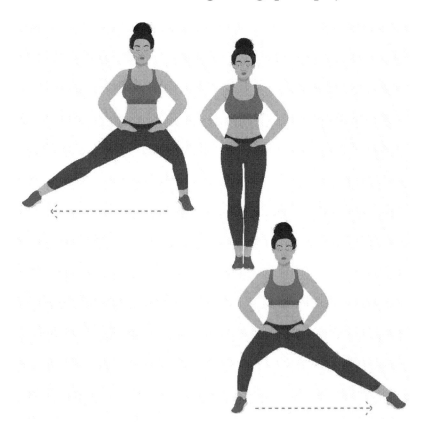

Instructions:

1. Stand tall with your feet hip-width apart.
2. Take a wide step out to your right while bending your right knee as far as you can without rounding your back.

3. Keep both feet flat on the floor.
4. Push through your right foot to return to standing.
5. Repeat on your left side.

Tip: Point your knees in the same direction as your feet.

Easier Option: Step out to the side without bending your knee.

Harder Option: Hold a weight close to your chest.

50. Weighted Lunges

Weighted lunges help develop your single-leg strength and stability. They work your glutes, quads, calves, hamstrings, and core. Weighted lunges add greater resistance to make the exercise more challenging.

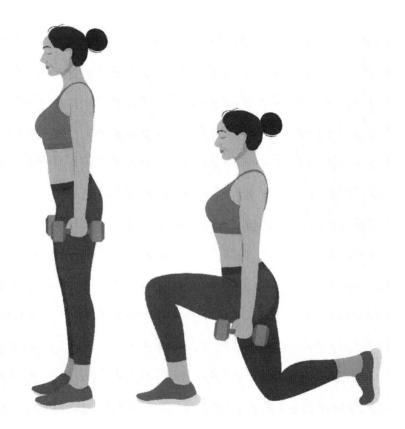

Instructions:

1. Stand tall with your feet hip-width apart and a weight in each hand at your side.
2. Pull your shoulder back, engage your core, and squeeze your buttock.

3. Take a step forward with your right foot while keeping your left foot planted.
4. Bend your right leg until it creates a 90-degree angle at the knee.
5. Keeping the weight in your front heel, push through the floor and lower the weight to come back to your starting position.
6. Perform half the repetitions on one side and the remaining on the opposite side.

Tip: Ensure your knees are pushed out during extension of the front leg. They should not be caving in.

Easier Option: Perform the exercise without the weight.

Harder Option: Remain in the split stance position rather than returning to standing between each repetition.

51. Weighted Squats

Weighted squats work your leg muscles, including the glutes, quads, hamstrings, calves, and core. Similar to regular air squats, but with added resistance to enhance strength benefits.

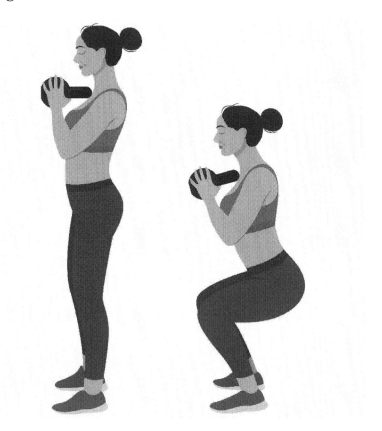

Instructions:

1. To perform weighted squats, stand with your feet shoulder-width apart.
2. Hold a weight against your chest.
3. Push your hips back and bend the knees until your buttock is lower than your knees.

4. Keep your back straight and core engaged throughout.
5. Drive through your midfoot to return to standing.
6. During extension, push your knees out.

Tip: Point your toes slightly out.

Easier Option: Perform the exercise without weight.

Harder Option: Hold a weight in each hand.

52. Clams

Clams build strength in the glutes, inner, and outer thighs. Your glutes play a significant role in stabilizing your pelvis therefore, it's important we keep it strong.

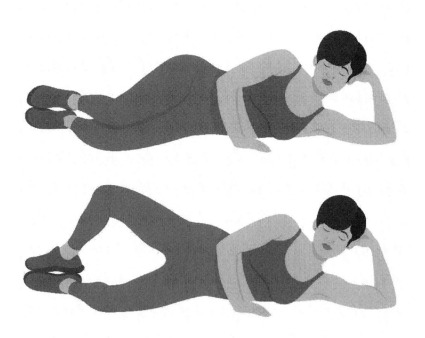

Instructions:

1. Begin lying on your left side with your hips and shoulders aligned.
2. Bend your knees slightly and prop your head up with your hand.
3. Brace your core and tuck your belly button in.

4. Keeping your toes together, rotate your right knee as far as you can without breaking hip alignment.
5. Pause for two seconds before returning to the starting position.

Tip: Keep your neck still.

Easier Option: Reduce the range of motion.

Harder Option: Wrap a resistance band just above your knees.

53. Leg Abduction

Leg abduction is a common everyday movement. We perform abduction when we step to the side or get out of bed. Leg abductions strengthen the hips and glutes.

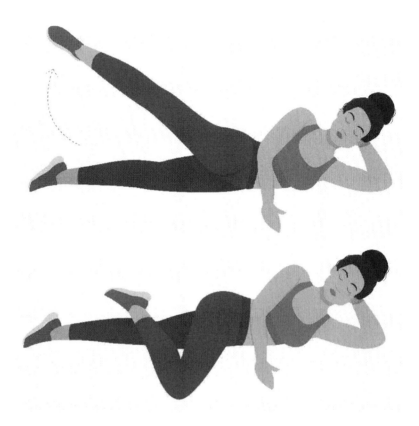

Instructions:

1. Begin lying on your right side with your legs extended and right arm propping your torso up.
2. Squeeze your core and buttock.
3. Lift your left leg away from your body as far as you comfortably can.
4. Hold for two seconds before slowly lowering.

5. Perform half the repetitions on your left leg and half on your right.

Tip: Keep your hips square.

Easier Option: Slightly bend your legs.

Harder Option: Place a resistance band just above your knees.

54. Cossack Squat

Cossack squats build strength in your legs and core while focusing on your inner thighs. Cossack squats also improve your posture by working the stabilizer muscles in your hips.

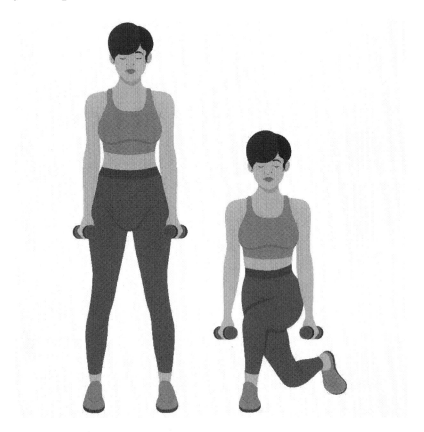

Instructions:

1. Stand tall with your feet hip-width apart with a weight in each hand at your sides.
2. Take a big step behind your left leg.
3. Bend your right knee and hips until your knee touches the floor.

4. Keep your back straight, core engaged, and buttock squeezed.
5. Push through your left leg to return to the starting position.
6. Perform half the reps on your right leg and half on your left.

Tip: Keep your front knee in line with your front knee.

Easier Option: Perform the exercise without weight.

Harder Option: Don't let your knee touch the floor, stop an inch above.

55. Standing Toe Touches

Standing toe touches are a great exercise to improve your mobility, core, and leg strength. It predominantly works your obliques and hamstrings.

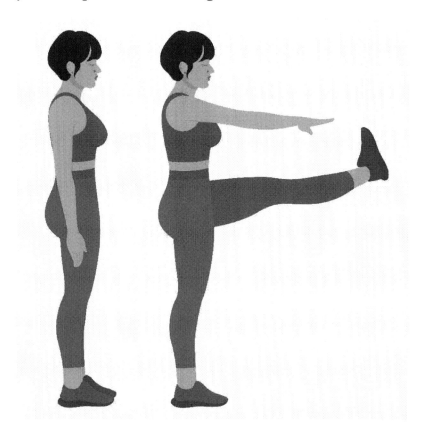

Instructions:

1. Stand tall with your feet shoulder-width apart.
2. Keeping your legs straight, raise your right leg in front of you as far as you comfortably can.
3. Meanwhile, raise your left arm to meet the toe.
4. Slowly lower and repeat on your opposite side.

Tip: Keep your core and glutes tight.

Easier Option: Bend your knees slightly.

Harder Option: Hold a weight in each hand.

56. Wall Assisted Single Leg Toe Touches

Wall assisted single leg toe touches work legs, core, and shoulder strength. They also develop single-leg balance, strength, stabilization, mobility, and posture.

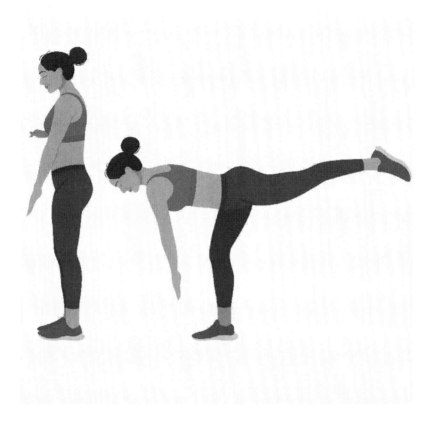

Instructions:

1. Stand tall with your feet hip-width apart.
2. Keep your left hand extended at your side and your right hand on a wall.
3. Pull your shoulder blades together and engage your core and buttock.

4. Slightly bend at the knees and raise your left foot off the floor, keeping your knees aligned.
5. From here, send the hips back without bending the knees. Keep your back flat, chest raised, and leg extended.
6. Lower your hand towards your toes as far as you can without rounding your back.
7. When you've reached maximal depth, push the hips forward to return to standing.
8. Repeat half the reps on one leg, then half on the opposite leg.

Tip: Pause between repetitions to regain your balance.

Easier Option: Place more weight onto the wall.

Harder Option: Add a weight.

57. Donkey Kicks

Donkey kicks work your core and glute muscles to build strength and stability.

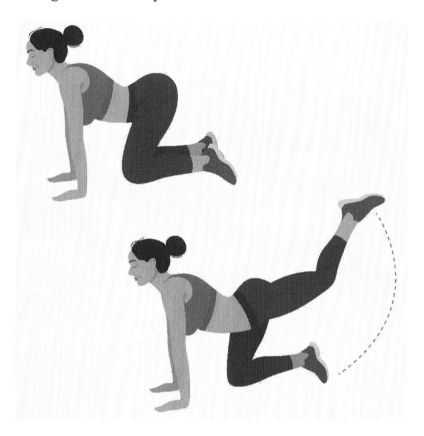

Instructions:

1. Start on your hand and knees.
2. Your hands should be directly under your shoulders and your knees under your hips.
3. Keep your back flat, core engaged, and glutes tensed.
4. Keeping your leg bent, raise your right leg until your thigh is in line with your torso.

5. Pause for one second before lowering to the starting position.
6. Repeat the movement on your left leg.

Tip: Keep your hips squared. Avoid any torso rotation.

Easier Option: Reduce the range of motion.

Harder Option: Place a resistance band above your knees.

58. Knee to Chest

Knee to chests improve your mobility, core, and leg strength. They work your hip flexors, abdominals, and quads.

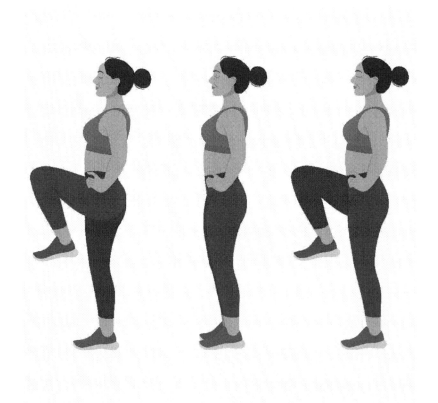

Instructions:

1. Stand tall with your feet shoulder-width apart.
2. Squeeze your core and glutes while pulling your shoulder blades together.
3. Bring your right knee to your chest, briefly hold, then lower.
4. Repeat on your left leg.

Tip: Look at a spot on the floor to help you balance.

Easier Option: Perform the movement seated.

Harder Option: Hold at the top of the movement for four seconds.

<u>59. Knee to Chest Box Step Up</u>

Knee to chest box step ups are an advanced version of the knee to chests. They improve your mobility, core, and leg strength. The additional step up places more emphasis on your glutes.

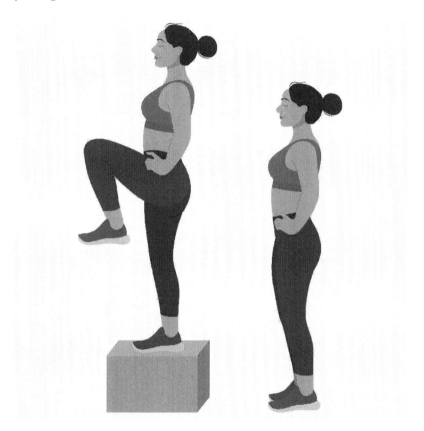

Instructions:

1. Stand tall with your feet shoulder-width apart.
2. Squeeze your core and glutes while pulling your shoulder blades together.
3. Place your right foot on the box.

4. Drive through your right foot to extend your leg and bring your left foot onto the box.
5. Slowly step down with your left foot, followed by your right leg.
6. Repeat on your opposite side.

Tip: Keep your leading knee pushed out.

Easier Option: Perform regular knee to chests.

Harder Option: Hold a weight in each hand.

60. Plié Squat

The plié squat strengthens the quads, hamstrings, glutes, and calves while increasing the range of motion in your hips.

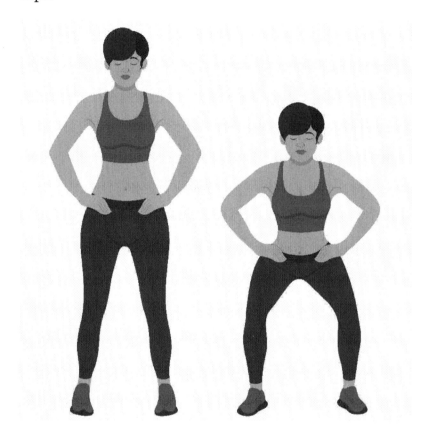

Instructions:

1. Stand with your feet outside shoulder-width apart.
2. Rotate your feet out to a 45-degree angle.
3. Put your hands on your hips.
4. Push your hips back and bend the knees until your buttock is just above knee height.

5. Keep your back straight and core engaged throughout.
6. Drive through your midfoot to return to standing.
7. During extension, push your knees out.

Tip: Keep your chest up.

Easier Option: Perform a wide squat.

Harder Option: Place a resistance band just above your knees.

Core Exercises

Contrary to popular belief, your core muscles aren't only your "6-pack". Your core includes your lower back, side, and deeper core muscles. The core muscles work together to provide stability and strength.

61. Cat Cow

The cat cow is a mobility exercise used to improve posture and balance. It also helps you relax while relieving stress.

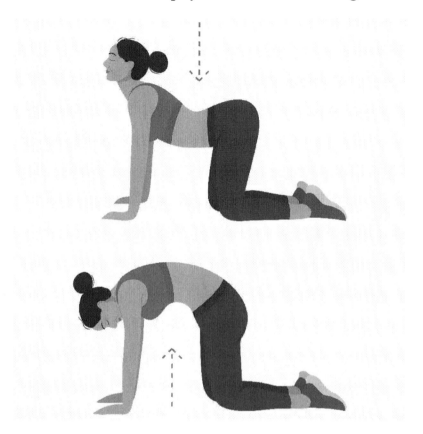

Instructions:

1. Start on your hands and knees with your hips over your knees and shoulders over your hands.
2. From here, lower your chest without bending your arms.
3. Then, bring your upper back up towards the ceiling, rounding your shoulders.

Tip: Imagine a piece of string is attached to your chest, and someone is pulling it towards the floor and ceiling.

Easier Option: Perform the movement in a chair.

Harder Option: Work through the two positions in one fluid movement.

62. V-Ups

V-ups work your core muscles to help build strength. V-ups are unique as they target the upper and lower abdomen due to both the arms and legs being involved. Apart from the abdomen, v-ups the obliques, back, quads, and hamstrings.

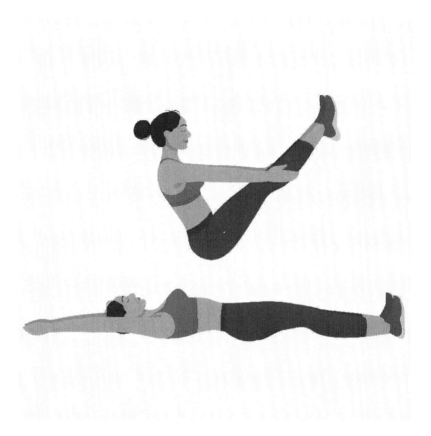

Instructions:

1. Begin lying face-up on the floor with your arms above your head and legs fully extended.

2. Keeping your arms and legs extended, simultaneously bring them towards each other, so they meet above your stomach.
3. Pause for a second before lowering to the floor.
4. Keep your core tight and lower back pressed into the floor throughout the movement.

Tip: Imagine your arms and legs are being pulled together.

Easier Option: Raise your legs and then your arms instead of performing the movement simultaneously.

Harder Option: During the lowering phase, pause just before your arms and legs touch the floor, then go straight into the next repetition.

63. Dead Bug

Dead bugs are a core exercise to help develop your core strength, coordination, and balance. They're great for strengthening the smaller muscles in your shoulders and hips too.

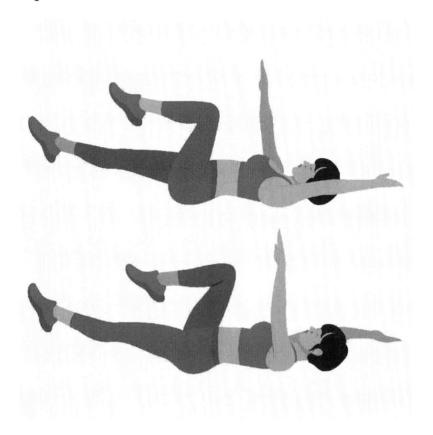

Instructions:

1. To perform the dead bug, begin by lying face-up on a mat.
2. Bring your knees towards your chest at a 90-degree angle and extend your arms towards the ceiling.

3. Slowly lower your right arm and left leg towards the floor.
4. Stop about 1-inch above the floor, pause for a second, then return to the center before repeating on the other side.

Tip: Press your lower back into the floor to engage your core.

Easier Option: Only move your leg or arm, not both.

Harder Option: Hold a weight in your hands.

64. Bicycle Crunches

Bicycle crunches are predominantly a core exercise focusing on rotational strength. A strong core protects the spine and helps you perform better in everyday tasks. The extension of the legs also activates the hip muscles.

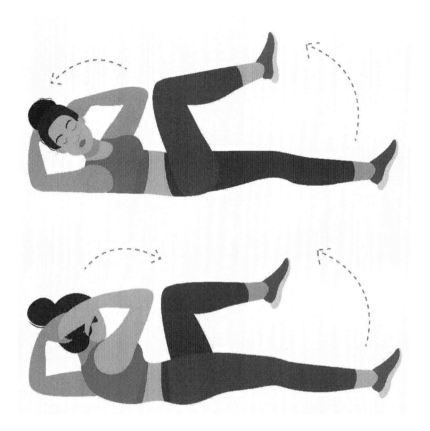

Instructions:

1. Start lying face-up on the floor with your legs fully extended.
2. Lift your feet off the floor until they are over your hips at a 90-degree angle.

3. Place your fingers on your temples and raise your upper back off the floor. This is your starting position.
4. Move your right elbow towards your left knee while simultaneously extending your right leg.
5. Return your arms and legs to the starting position before repeating the movement on the opposite side.

Tip: Do not pull your neck up.

Easier Option: Keep your upper back on the floor.

Harder Option: At the top of the movement, when your knee and elbow are touching, pause for two seconds.

65. Plank Hip Dips

Plank hip dips are a full-body exercise used to develop strength and stability. Plank hip dips build single-leg glute, core, and tricep strength.

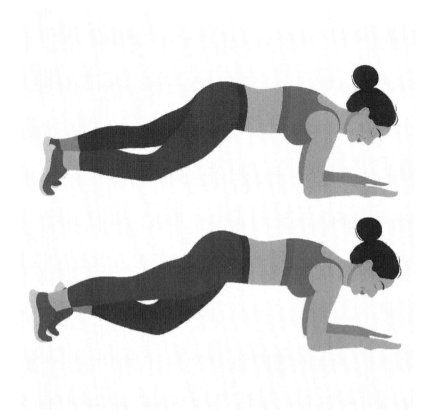

Instructions:

1. Begin sitting on the floor with your legs extended and torso upright.
2. Place your hands on the floor behind your shoulders.
3. Lean back, so your arms take the weight of your body.

4. Bring your feet to your buttock while remaining flat on the floor.
5. Push through your feet and palms to lift your hips slightly off the floor.
6. From here, fully extend your left leg towards the sky.
7. Pause for one second, then lower back to the floor. Repeat the movement on your right leg.
8. Continue alternating.

Tip: Squeeze your core and buttock throughout.

Easier Option: Keep your buttock on the floor.

Harder Option: Lift your hips with each extension.

66. Side Plank

Side planks build strength and stability in the core and shoulder muscles. Placing your weight on alternate sides of the body helps develop single joint strength.

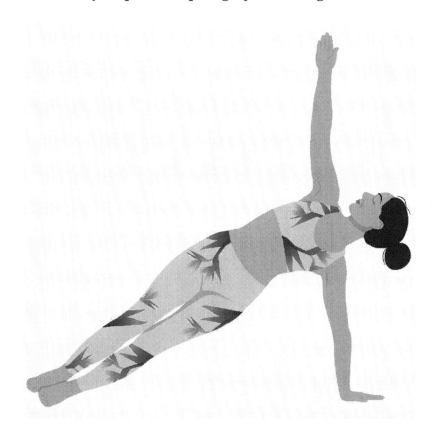

Instructions:

1. Begin lying on your right side with your legs extended and right arm propping your torso up.
2. Lift your hips off the floor.
3. Your shoulders, buttock, and ankles should all be aligned.
4. Squeeze your core and buttock.

5. Hold this position for half the time, then switch side.

Tip: Raise your opposite hand towards the sky.

Easier Option: Keep your knees on the floor.

Harder Option: Hold a weight in your hand.

67. Low Plank Knee to Floor

The low plank knee to floor improves full-body stability and strengthens your spine, back, core, glutes, hamstrings, shoulders, and triceps. Movement at the knees puts greater emphasis on your hip flexors.

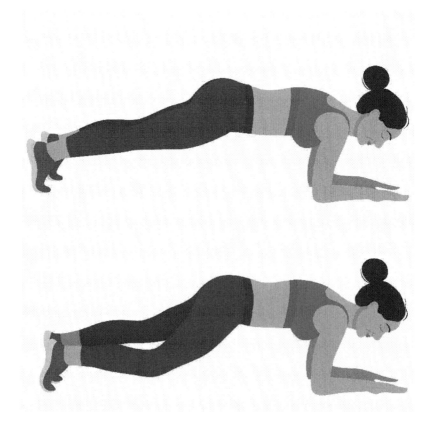

Instructions:

1. Start in the low plank position.
2. Place your elbows under your shoulders and toes on the floor.
3. Your shoulders, buttock, and ankles should all be aligned.

4. Squeeze your core and buttock.
5. Lower your right knee to the floor, pause for one second, then return to the starting position.
6. Repeat this movement on your left side.

Tip: Avoid any rotation by keeping your core tight and facing the floor.

Easier Option: Hold a low plank position without moving your knees.

Harder Option: Come up to a full plank position on your hands.

68. Plank Tucks

Plank tucks strengthen your core and cardiovascular system. They also help build strength in the shoulders, glutes, quads, hamstrings, and triceps.

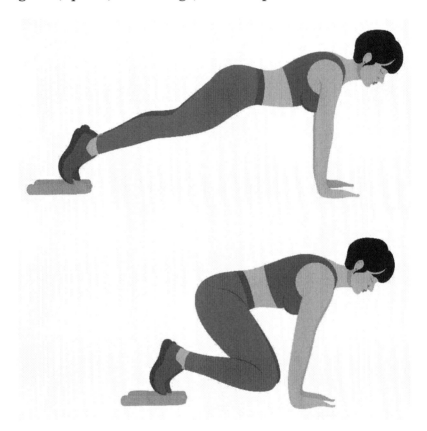

Instructions:

1. Start in the plank position.
2. Place a towel underneath your feet (on a slippery surface).
3. Place your hands under your shoulders and toes on the floor.

4. Your shoulders, buttock, and ankles should all be aligned.
5. Squeeze your core and buttock.
6. Pull your feet to your buttock.
7. Briefly pause before sliding back to the plank position.

Tip: Squeeze your legs together to reduce the instability.

Easier Option: Perform plank hops if you cannot perform this movement.

Harder Option: Pause at the top of the tuck for three seconds.

69. Plank Rotation

Plank rotations strengthen your core, balance, and stability. They also build strength in your back, core, glutes, hamstrings, shoulders, and triceps.

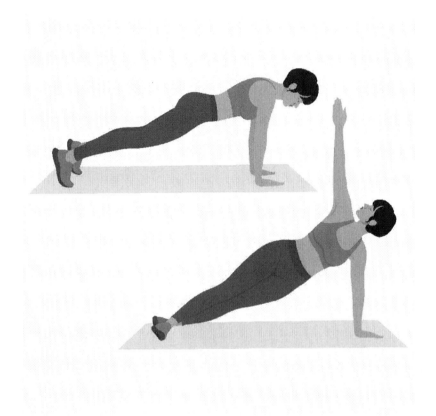

Instructions:

1. Start in the plank position.
2. Place your hands under your shoulders and toes on the floor.
3. Your shoulders, buttock, and ankles should all be aligned.
4. Squeeze your core and buttock.

5. Lift your right hand off the floor and twist your torso towards the sky.
6. Hold for 2 seconds before internally rotating your torso back to the center.
7. Perform half the repetitions on your right side before switching to the left.

Tip: Always look in the same direction as your hand is moving.

Easier Option: Perform the exercise on your knees.

Harder Option: Hold a weight in your hand.

70. Sprinter Sit Ups

Sprinter sit ups strengthen your abdominals and obliques. They also help build core and rotational stability.

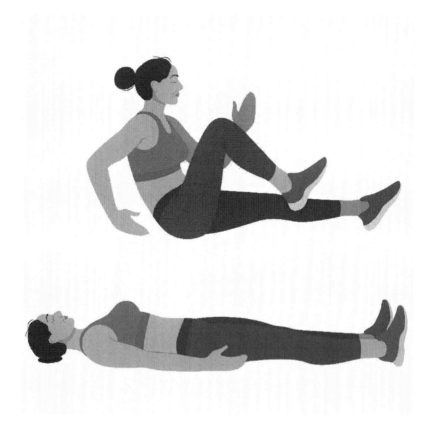

Instructions:

1. Begin lying on the floor with your legs extended and arms at your side.
2. Press your lower back into the floor while lifting your shoulder blades and feet off the ground.
3. Drive your left elbow to your right knee, pause for one second, then slowly lower to the starting position.

4. Repeat the movement on your opposite side.

Tip: Keep your back straight and stable throughout.

Easier Option: Only crunch your knees, not your arms.

Harder Option: Hold a weight in each hand.

71. Hollow Archs

Hollow archs help build a strong and stable core. They target the abdominals, diaphragm, hip flexors, and core. They are also beneficial for improving your posture.

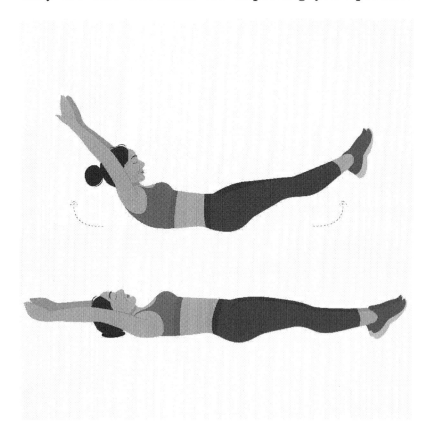

Instructions:

1. Begin lying on the floor with your legs extended and your arms above your head.
2. Push your shoulders, upper back, and lower back into the floor while squeezing your core.
3. Squeeze your ankles together and arms to your ears.

4. Lift your upper back and feet off the floor until you feel your abs tense.
5. Hold for a second before slowly lowering.

Tip: Keep your lower back pressed into the floor through the exercise.

Easier Option: Only raise your feet, not your upper back.

Harder Option: Hold a weight in each hand.

72. Leg Raises

Leg raises build your core strength and stability. Leg raises focus on the lower part of your abdominals which can be difficult to target.

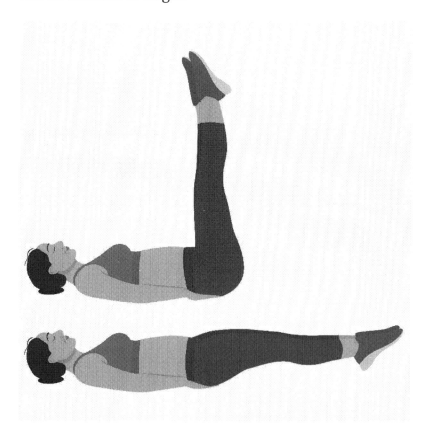

Instructions:

1. Begin lying on the floor with your legs extended and arms at your side.
2. Push your shoulders, upper back, and lower back into the floor while squeezing your core.
3. Squeeze your ankles together.
4. Lift your feet off the floor to a 90-degree angle.

5. Hold for a second before slowly lowering.

Tip: Control the movement, don't rely on momentum.

Easier Option: Bend your legs to a 90-degree angle.

Harder Option: Do not lower your legs to the floor. Pause an inch from the floor before performing the next repetition.

73. Leg Raise with Clap

Leg raise with clap is an advanced version of a regular leg raise. It builds core strength and stability. However, the clap portion targets the upper part of your abdominals. Therefore, it's a great full abdominal exercise.

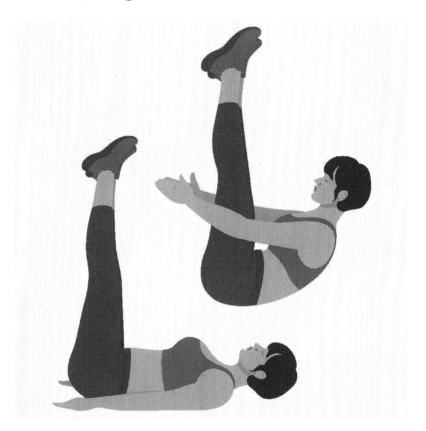

Instructions:

1. Begin lying on the floor with your legs extended and arms at your side.
2. Push your shoulders, upper back, and lower back into the floor while squeezing your core.
3. Squeeze your ankles together.

4. Lift your feet off the floor to a 90-degree angle.
5. Lift your upper back off the floor perform a clap behind your knees.
6. Slowly lower your upper back and legs back to the floor.

Tip: Keep your hands at your sides.

Easier Option: Bend your legs to a 90-degree angle.

Harder Option: Raise your feet and upper back simultaneously.

74. Alternating Superman

The alternating superman exercise is an advanced version of regular supermans. It works single limb strength and stability in your upper back, lower back, glutes, hamstrings, and core. It's a great exercise for improving posture and alleviating back pain.

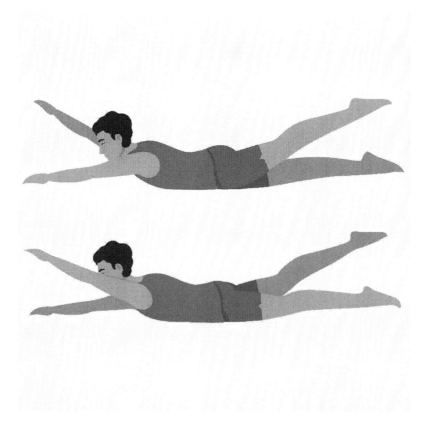

Instructions:

1. Begin lying face down with your legs extended and arms above your head.
2. Push your hips into the floor while squeezing your core and buttocks.

3. Lift your right arm and left foot off the floor as far as you comfortably can.
4. Hold for two seconds before slowly lowering and repeating on the opposite side.

Tip: Think of the action like a front crawl.

Easier Option: Bend your arms to a 90-degree angle.

Harder Option: Hold a weight in each hand.

75. Flutter Kicks

Flutter kicks strengthen your core by targeting the lower abdominal and hip flexors.

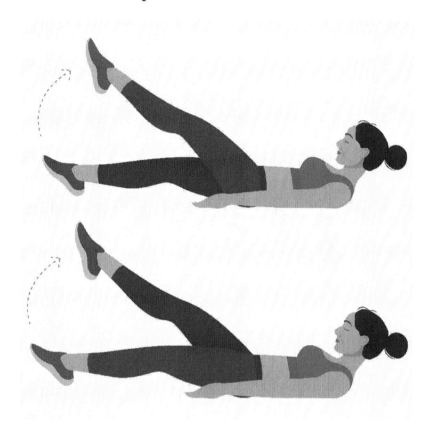

Instructions:

1. Begin lying on the floor with your legs extended and arms at your side.
2. Push your shoulders, upper back, and lower back into the floor while squeezing your core.
3. Lift your feet 5-inches off the floor while keeping your lower back pressed into the floor.

4. Cross your feet over each other - like a scissor action.

Tip: Control the movement, don't be tempted to go fast.

Easier Option: Raise your feet higher.

Harder Option: Lift your upper back off the floor during the movement.

76. Roll Outs

Roll outs build strength in the core, specifically the abdominals, obliques, and lower back. Roll outs also work your shoulders, upper back, and hamstrings.

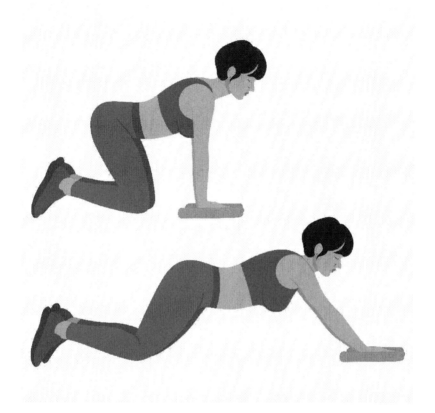

Instructions:

1. Begin kneeling on the floor with your feet together.
2. Place your hands on a towel (on a slippery surface) with your hands directly under your shoulders.
3. Squeeze your core and buttock while drawing your shoulder blades back.

4. Push your hands forward while keeping your back straight and core engaged.
5. Lower your chest to the floor as far as you can without breaking form.
6. Pause for a second, then return to an upright position.

Tip: Don't push your hands into the floor.

Easier Option: Reduce the range of motion.

Harder Option: Take your knees off the floor and come onto your toes.

77. Tuck Ups

Tuck ups help build a strong and stable core. They target the abdominals, diaphragm, lower back, hip flexors, and core.

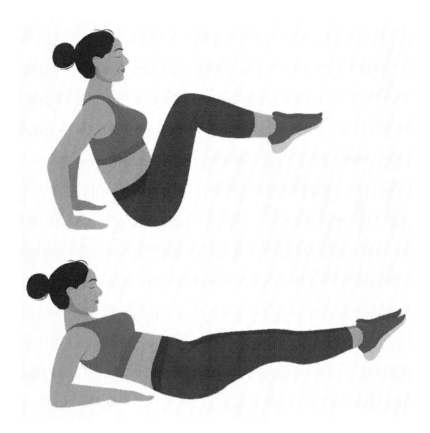

Instructions:

1. Begin sitting on the floor with your legs bent.
2. Place your hands flat on the floor just behind your hips.
3. Lean back to push the weight onto your hands.
4. Lift your knees to your chest.
5. Engage your core - this is your starting position.

6. Extend your legs while simultaneously shifting your weight onto your forearms.
7. Pause for a second before returning to the starting position.

Tip: Keep your neck in a neutral position.

Easier Option: Only extend your legs, do not come onto your forearms.

Harder Option: Perform single-leg tucks.

78. Alternating Knee Touches

Alternating knee touches build strength in your core, lower back, upper back, hip flexors, quads, and shoulders. The rotational movement also puts great emphasis on your obliques.

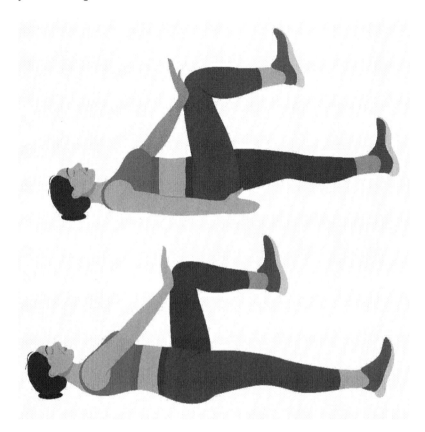

Instructions:

1. Begin lying on the floor with your legs extended and arms at your side.
2. Push your shoulders, upper back, and lower back into the floor while squeezing your core.

3. Bend your right knee to a 90-degree angle. Touch your right knee with your left hand.
4. Slowly lower your leg back to the floor before repeating on your left leg.

Tip: Keep your lower back pushed into the ground.

Easier Option: Only move your legs, not your arms.

Harder Option: Lift your upper back off the floor with each knee touch.

79. Hip Lifts

Hip lifts are a core exercise targeting your lower abdominals. They are also a great exercise for building lower back strength.

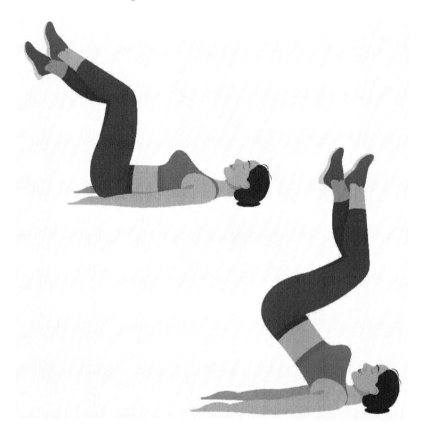

Instructions:

1. Begin lying on your back with your arms at your side and legs bent to a 90-degree angle.
2. Engage your core and push your lower back into the floor.
3. Lift your legs towards the sky, then control the descent to return to the starting position.

Tip: Imagine you're trying to touch the sky with your toes.

Easier Option: Return your feet to the floor after each repetition.

Harder Option: Control the descent for a three-second count.

80. Russian Twists

Russian twists help develop rotational core strength. They work your obliques, abdominals, and lower back.

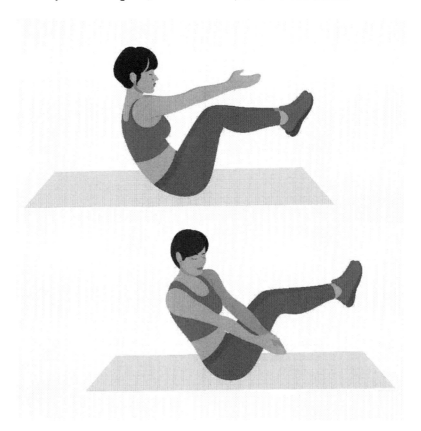

Instructions:

1. Begin sitting on the floor with your torso upright and feet flat.
2. Lean slightly back before lifting your feet off the floor.
3. Keep your core tight and chest up.
4. Rotate both arms to the right, touch the floor, then return to the center.

5. Repeat on your left side.

Tip: Keep your head in a neutral position.

Easier Option: Keep your feet on the floor.

Harder Option: Hold a weight.

Mobility Exercises

While not a specific area of strength, good mobility is an essential part of a healthy life. Mobility is linked to joint health, flexibility, and stability.

81. Plank to Down Dog

Plank to down dog helps develop your core strength and mobility. Additionally, it will help improve stability and strength in your spine, back, core, glutes, hamstrings, shoulders, and triceps.

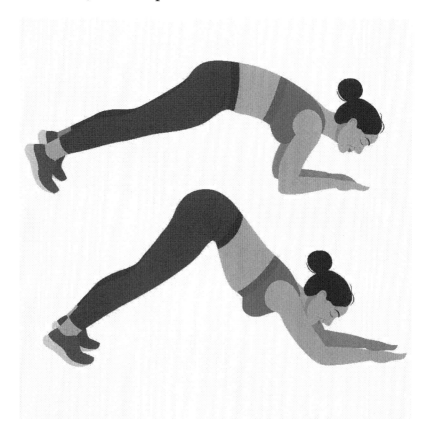

Instructions:

1. Start in the plank position.
2. Place your hands under your shoulders and toes on the floor.
3. Your shoulders, buttock, and ankles should all be aligned.

4. Squeeze your core and buttock.
5. Push your hips back into an upside-down v position - this is the down dog position.
6. Hold for two seconds before returning to the plank position.
7. Continue moving through these two positions.

Tip: Push away with your arms as you tuck your head through.

Easier Option: Hold the down dog position.

Harder Option: Perform a press up at the end of each down dog.

82. Pigeon

The pigeon stretch improves mobility and flexibility in your hips. It stretches the muscles in your quads, hamstrings, back, hip flexors, and groin. The pigeon can also help improve your posture after a long day of sitting.

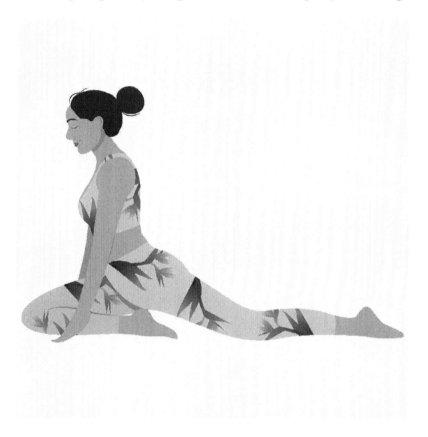

Instructions:

1. Start in the plank position.
2. Place your hands under your shoulders and toes on the floor.
3. Your shoulders, buttock, and ankles should all be aligned.

4. Squeeze your core and buttock.
5. Push your hips back into an upside-down v-position.
6. Step your right foot forward and place your right knee next to your right hand.
7. Let your left knee drop to the floor.
8. Drop your hips to the floor and bend over your right shin.
9. Repeat on your left leg.

Tip: Keep your hips square.

Easier Option: Place a block under your forearms.

Harder Option: Aim to bend your chest on the floor.

83. Dynamic Pigeon

The dynamic pigeon is a variation of the traditional pigeon. It improves mobility and flexibility in your hips. It also stretches the muscles in your quads, hamstrings, back, hip flexors, and groin. The dynamic element allows you to reach further in the stretch.

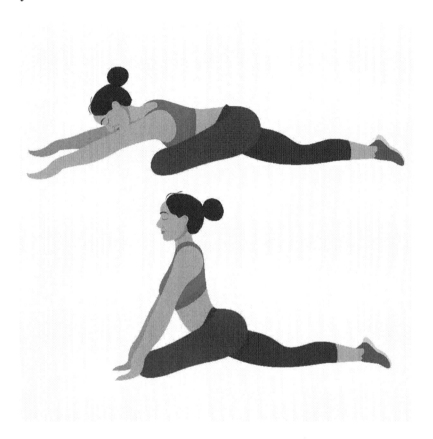

Instructions:

1. Start in the plank position.
2. Place your hands under your shoulders and toes on the floor.

3. Your shoulders, buttock, and ankles should all be aligned.
4. Squeeze your core and buttock.
5. Push your hips back into an upside-down v position.
6. Step your right foot forward and place your right knee next to your right hand.
7. Let your left knee drop to the floor.
8. Drop your hips to the floor and bend over your right shin.
9. Hold the bend for two seconds before raising your torso upright.
10. Repeat on your left leg.

Tip: Use a block to support your bent knee.

Easier Option: Perform the pigeon exercise.

Harder Option: Hold each bend for five seconds.

84. Cow

The cow is a yoga pose that stretches your torso and neck. It's a great way to improve your posture and spine health.

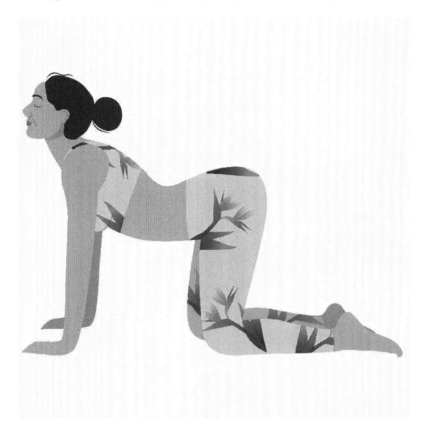

Instructions:

1. Begin on your hands and knees.
2. Ensure your hands are directly under your shoulders and knees under your hips.
3. Keep your head in a neutral position and squeeze your core.
4. Lift your chest while drawing the belly button down.

5. Hold this position.

Tip: Pull your shoulder blades apart and down.

Easier Option: Release the position every 10 seconds.

Harder Option: Perform the cat-cow exercise.

85. Seated Cat Pose

The seated cat pose stretches the lower back, core, chest, hips, and neck.

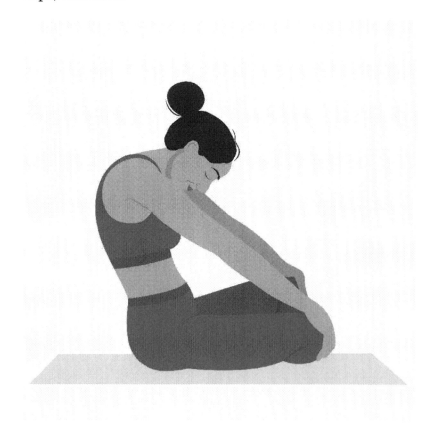

Instructions:

1. Begin sat on the floor with your legs crossed.
2. Place your palms on the outside of your knees.
3. Round your back and drop your chin to your chest.
4. Hold this position.

Tip: Pull your shoulder blades apart and down.

Easier Option: Perform the exercise in a chair.

Harder Option: Perform the exercise standing up.

86. Hero

The hero pose increases flexibility in your hips and knees while encouraging good hip, leg, and knee alignment. It also opens up the hips while stretching the quads.

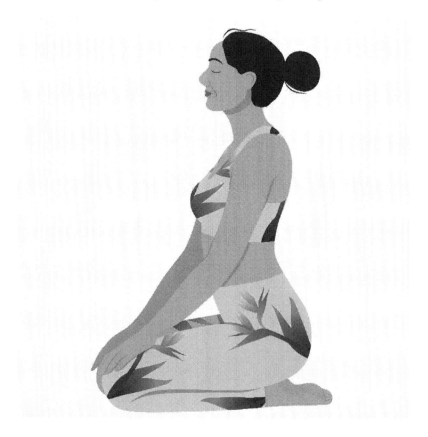

Instructions:

1. Begin kneeling with your shins flat on the floor and inner thighs touching.
2. Move your feet outside hip-width.
3. Sit back onto your heels and lean your torso slightly forward.
4. Hold this position.

Tip: Place your hands on your knees and push your chest up.

Easier Option: Place a folded blanket under your shins to add elevation.

Harder Option: Pull on your knees to enhance the back and shoulder stretch.

87. Extended Triangle

The extended triangle stretches your hips, groin, hamstrings, calves, shoulder, and chest.

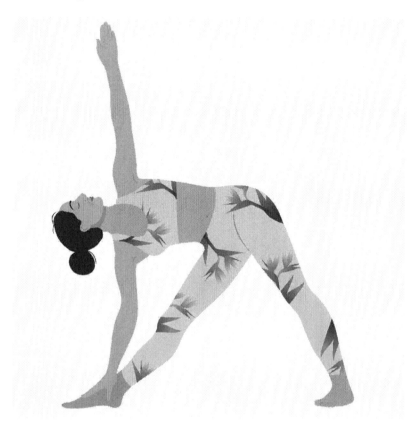

Instructions:

1. Stand with your feet just outside shoulder-width.
2. Extend your arms to the side until they are parallel to the floor.
3. Pull your shoulder blades together and rotate your palms down.
4. Rotate your right foot in while rotating your left foot to the side.

5. Bend at the hips to bring your left hand to your left foot.
6. Your right hand should be pointing to the sky.
7. Hold this position before repeating on the opposite side.

Tip: Look towards your hand in the sky.

Easier Option: Bend down as far as you can without rounding your back.

Harder Option: Step your feet out wider to enhance the groin stretch.

88. Superman

The superman exercise strengthens your upper back, lower back, glutes, hamstrings, and core. It's a great exercise for improving posture and alleviating back pain.

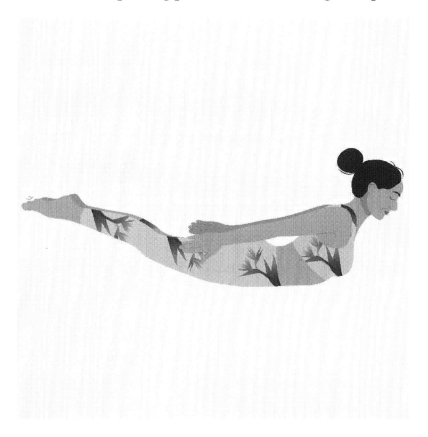

Instructions:

1. Begin lying face down with your legs extended and arms above your head.
2. Push your hips into the floor while squeezing your core and buttocks.
3. Lift your chest and feet off the floor as far as you comfortably can.

4. Hold for two seconds before slowly lowering.

Tip: Keep your hips pushed down.

Easier Option: Bend your arms to a 90-degree angle.

Harder Option: Hold a weight in each hand.

89. Downward Facing Dog

The downward facing dog strengthens the shoulder joint, back, calves, hamstrings, and forearms. It also opens up your hip and shoulder joints.

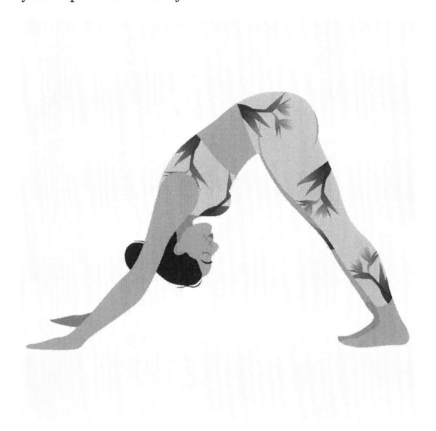

Instructions:

1. Start in the plank position.
2. Place your hands under your shoulders and toes on the floor.
3. Your shoulders, buttock, and ankles should all be aligned.
4. Squeeze your core and buttock.

5. Walk your hands back and lift your hips back into an upside-down v position.
6. Hold this position.

Tip: Keep your neck in a neutral position.

Easier Option: Perform the exercise on your knees.

Harder Option: Bend the elbows slightly.

90. Kneeling Prayer

The kneeling prayer increases flexibility in your hips and knees. It also strengthens your lower back and improves your balance.

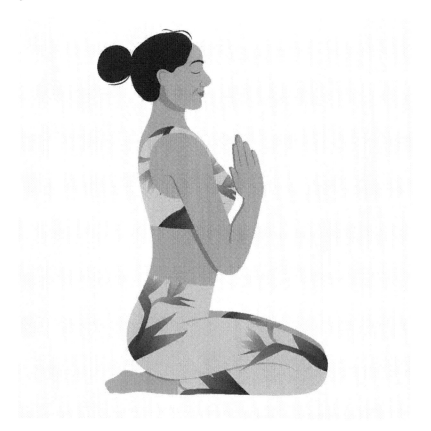

Instructions:

1. Stand tall with your feet together and hands in a prayer position.
2. Slowly fall to your knees while keeping your legs together.
3. Rest your buttock on your heels.

4. Tense your core and pull your shoulder blades together, so your torso is in an upright position.
5. Hold this position.

Tip: Practice deep breathing.

Easier Option: Use your hands to help lower yourself to the floor.

Harder Option: Drive your hips forward and hold the position with your thighs in line with your torso.

91. Crescent Lunge

The crescent lunge improves flexibility in your hips, groin, and shoulders.

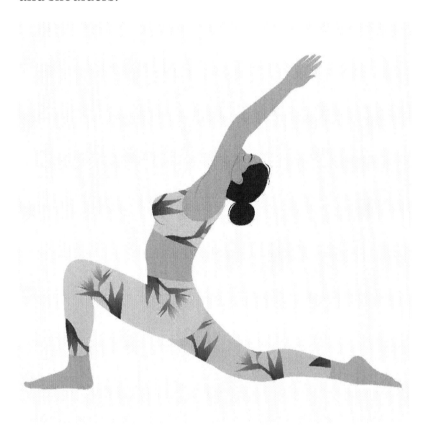

Instructions:

1. Begin standing tall with your feet shoulder-width apart.
2. Take a long step forward with your right foot while keeping your left foot planted.
3. Bend your right leg until it creates a 90-degree angle at the knee.

4. Ensure your shoulders are relaxed and your core is engaged.
5. Lower your hips and rest your back leg on the floor.
6. Extend your arm above your head and lean back.
7. Hold this position before repeating on the opposite leg.

Tip: Keep your hips square and pushed towards the floor.

Easier Option: Place a towel or block under your back foot.

Harder Option: Hold a weight in each hand.

92. Cobra

The cobra improves your posture and alleviates back pain by strengthening the shoulders, arms, and back muscles.

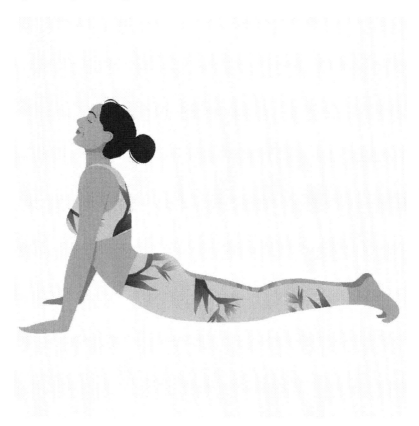

Instructions:

1. Begin lying on the floor face down.
2. Place your hands by your ribs and place your feet hip-width apart.
3. Push your feet and quads into the floor.
4. Push through your palms to raise your chest and head.

5. Keep your hips on the floor and pull your shoulder blades together.
6. Hold this position.

Tip: Keep a slight bend in your arms.

Easier Option: Place your forearms on the floor and don't fully extend your arms.

Harder Option: Rest your feet on a book or block to extend the stretch.

93. Sphinx

The sphinx strengthens your spine and glutes while stretching the chest, shoulders, and abdominals.

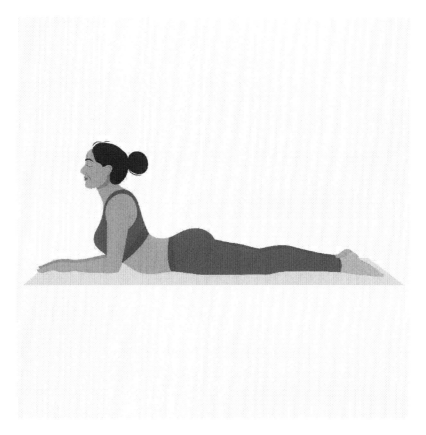

Instructions:

1. Begin lying on the floor face down.
2. Place your elbows under your shoulders and place your feet hip-width apart.
3. Push your feet and quads into the floor.
4. Push through your elbows to raise your chest and head.

5. Keep your hips on the floor and pull your shoulder blades together.
6. Hold this position.

Tip: Rotate your thighs inwards.

Easier Option: Place a rolled-up towel in a U-shape on the floor. Lie on the towel to support the lift.

Harder Option: Extend your arms fully.

94. Round Forward Fold

The round forward fold stretches your hamstrings and back while improving mobility in the hips and shoulders.

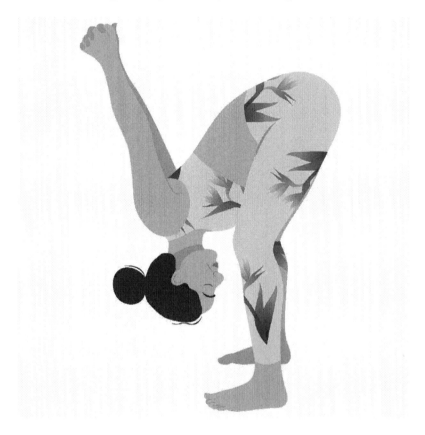

Instructions:

1. Stand tall with your feet hip-width apart.
2. Bend forward at the hips as far as you comfortably can.
3. Push your feet through the floor and lift your buttock towards the sky.
4. Keep your hips over your ankles.

5. Raise your arms above your head as far as you comfortably can.
6. Hold this position.

Tip: Push your knees out.

Easier Option: Bend your knees.

Harder Option: Hold a weight in each hand.

95. Baby Cobra

The baby cobra is a modified version of the cobra pose. It improves your posture and alleviates back pain by strengthening the shoulders, arms, and back muscles.

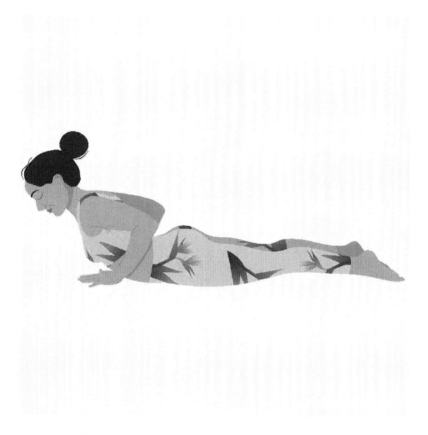

Instructions:

1. Begin lying on the floor face down.
2. Place your hands by your ribs and place your feet hip-width apart.
3. Push your feet and quads into the floor.
4. Keep your hips on the floor and pull your shoulder blades together.

5. Hold this position.

Tip: Your arms should not extend. Focus on stretching your shoulder blades rather than creating movement.

Easier Option: Hold the same position but do not force your shoulder blades to move.

Harder Option: Perform the full cobra.

96. Camel

The camel pose helps improve posture and back pain by strengthening the core, hip flexors, chest, shoulders, quads, hamstrings, back, and glutes.

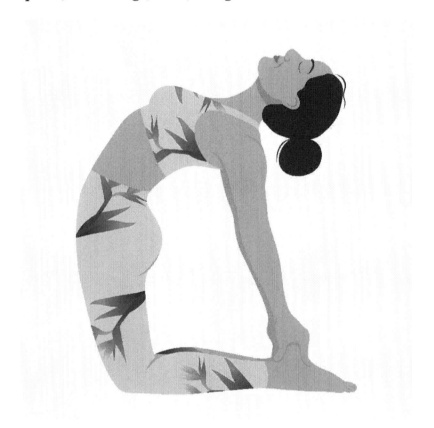

Instructions:

1. Begin on your knees with your shins flat on the floor and feet hip-width apart.
2. Push your feet into the floor.
3. Stack your hips directly over your knees.
4. Lift your chest and neck, then place your hands on your heels.

5. Push through with your hips.

Tip: Don't force the pose, slowly move into it.

Easier Option: Place your hands on your hips.

Harder Option: Place your hands behind your toes.

97. Bridge

The bridge can be used to alleviate knee and lower back pain by strengthening the glutes, core, lower back, hamstrings, and hips.

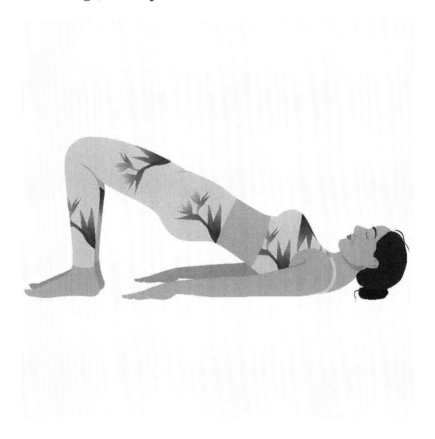

Instructions:

1. Begin lying on the floor with your legs extended and arms at your side.
2. Pull your feet to your buttock until they are flat on the floor.
3. Push your shoulders, upper back, and lower back into the floor while squeezing your core.

4. Engage your glutes, then push your hips towards the sky.
5. At the top of the movement, your knees, hips, and shoulders should be aligned.
6. Hold this position.

Tip: Imagine your pelvis is being pulled by a piece of string from the sky.

Easier Option: Place your feet further from your core.

Harder Option: Place a weight on your groin area.

98. Standing Forward Bend

The standing forward bend stretches your hamstrings and back while improving mobility in the hips and shoulders.

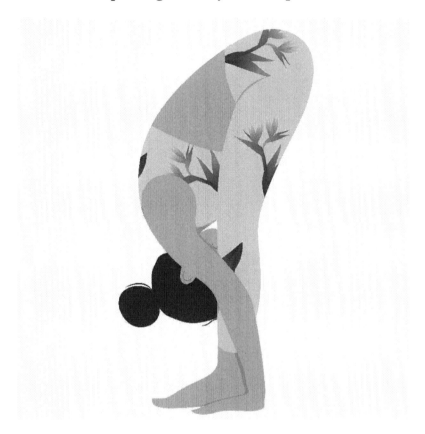

Instructions:

1. Stand tall with your feet hip-width apart.
2. Bend forward at the hips as far as you comfortably can.
3. Push your feet through the floor and lift your buttock towards the sky.
4. Keep your hips over your ankles.
5. Hold this position.

Tip: Push your knees out.

Easier Option: Bend your knees.

Harder Option: Place your palms behind your feet.

99. Boat

The boat pose develops core strength and stability in the back and abdomen. Specifically, it strengthens the abdominals, hip flexors, and spine.

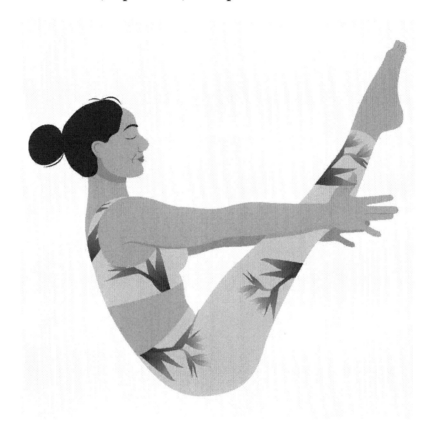

Instructions:

1. Begin seated with your knees bent and your feet flat on the floor.
2. Place your hands next to your hips.
3. Keeping your back straight, lean your torso back while lifting your feet off the floor.
4. Extend your legs and push your chest up.

5. Extend your arms forwards off the floor while maintaining a tight core.
6. Your body should now be in a V-shape.
7. Hold this position.

Tip: Spread your shoulder blades apart.

Easier Option: Bend your knees and keep your hands on the floor.

Harder Option: Lower your feet to an inch off the floor, then raise them back up to work the lower abdomen harder.

<u>100. Reverse Warrior Pose</u>

The reverse warrior pose strengthens the muscles in the legs and improves your hip and shoulder mobility.

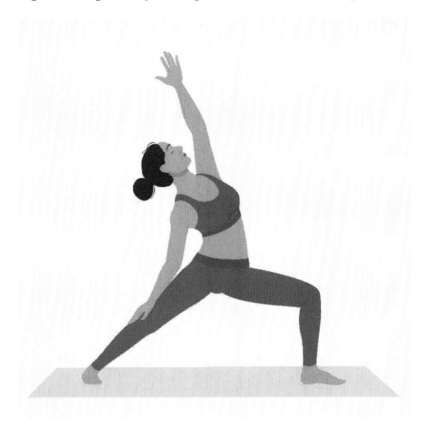

Instructions:

1. Stand with your feet just outside shoulder-width.
2. Extend your arms to the side until they are parallel to the floor.
3. Pull your shoulder blades together and rotate your palms down.
4. Lift your right arm towards the ceiling while touching your left toes with your left hand.

5. Your gaze should follow your right hand.
6. Keep your back straight and core engaged.
7. Hold this position for a few seconds, then repeat on the opposite side.

Tip: Focus on lifting your chest.

Easier Option: Gaze at your foot to take some pressure off your neck.

Harder Option: Hold a weight in each hand.

Part 4: 12 Weeks of Strength Training

Over the next 12 weeks, you'll be undergoing a strength training program to improve your strength and overall health.

The following strength program is based on the idea of progressive overload. What do we mean by the term "progressive overload"? Put simply, the fitter we get, the more we'll do. To continue getting stronger and fitter, we must continue to work the body harder. If we keep doing the same thing, our progress will come to a halt.

This program can be performed by all abilities, from beginners to advanced. Of course, everyone is different, and we all have our capabilities and areas to improve on. That's why we've designed this program to suit your current abilities. Throughout the program, you'll see options for an easier or harder version of the exercise. Therefore, you can follow through with the program while remaining within your individual limits.

Please read the whole section before your first workout to ensure you're comfortable with what each session will entail.

How to Use the Program

The following 12-week strength training program has been divided into three phases:

- Phase 1: Weeks 1-4 Beginner Level
- Phase 2: Weeks 5-8 Intermediate Level
- Phase 3: Weeks 9-12 Advanced Level

Each phase will build upon the phase prior, to ensure we're making continuous improvements. During phase one, you'll perform two workouts a week, then moving up to three days a week in phases two and three.

When you perform, these sessions are entirely up to you, although we do recommend taking one day off after each session. This is to help the body recover optimally, so we're not limited by fatigue in our next session.

Each workout will follow a similar format but will get progressively harder. All workouts have been designed to strengthen the entire body. In other plans, you might have seen workouts are split into body parts such as legs on one day and back and arms on another. This is a great split for people who work out 5-6 times a week but isn't the best option for those looking to get stronger for everyday life. For example, imagine picking an object off the floor and placing it on a shelf. This kind of everyday movement requires full-body strength. Therefore, if we want to improve our lives, we must train in a similar way. That's why we prefer to implement full-body workouts into our program.

Let's take a look at a typical session:

Exercise	Reps	Sets	Rest
Air Squats	10-15	2	90 Seconds
Tricep Dips	10-15	2	90 Seconds
Swimmers	10-15	2	90 Seconds
Glute Bridge	10-15	2	90 Seconds
Press Ups	10-15	2	90 Seconds
Dead Bug	10-15	2	90 Seconds
Standing Toe Touches	10-15	2	90 Seconds
Cat Cow	10-15	2	90 Seconds

As you can see there are eight exercises. Exercises can be further divided into multi-joint, upper body, lower body, core, and mobility. Performing exercises from each category helps us build strength in the key areas of the body for improved functional fitness.

Each session will have the following terms:

- Exercise: movement you will be performing
- Reps: number of times you will be performing the exercise
- Sets: number of times you repeat the allocated reps
- Rest: time spent resting between sets and reps

235

For the workout above, I would perform 10-15 air squats then take a 90-second break. I would then perform another 10-15 air squats twice, with a 90 seconds break in between. Once I finished my 3rd set of squats, I would rest for 90 seconds before repeating this sequence for the tricep dips and so on.

Some exercises will mention the use of an "odd object". We will use "odd objects" to provide external resistance to help build your strength. An "odd object" can be a piece of gym equipment such as a dumbbell, barbell, kettlebell, or resistance band, but don't worry if you haven't got any of these things. Everyday household items can work just as well. Use cans of food, water bottles, or a backpack full of books. Throughout the program, you will aim to increase the weight for each movement. If exercising with weight sounds a bit too much right now, that's also fine. I recommend starting without any weight and just going through the correct movement pattern. Building good movement patterns will get your muscles used to the motion and strengthen the stabilizer muscles around the joint. Over time, you will get comfortable with the movement, and that's when you'll add in weight.

When should you increase the weight? Weight should be added when you're performing the movement proficiently for more than the assigned reps. Take the example workout; if you can perform 20 reps without any weight AND perform the correct technique, then you should add weight. If you can only perform 4 reps with a heavy weight or are moving with bad technique, that's a sign to lower the weight. The aim is to find a weight you can perform 10-15 good reps with.

Other plans will suggest increasing weight by a specific number each week, but this approach doesn't take into account individual variability. For example, if your training has been going well you might be able to lift significantly more than the recommended weight. On the other hand, if you're having a less than desirable session, your body might not be able to cope with the added weight just yet. Therefore, we believe it's much more effective to listen to our bodies and let them tell us when and when they can't take the progression.

How to Go from One Level to the Other

We've mentioned everyone progresses at different rates, which is fine. This program has been designed to progress each week; therefore, it assumes your progression will be linear. However, we might not always be ready for the next phase of training. Again, it's okay. If you don't feel physically ready to progress onto the next phase, repeat some or all of the previous phase until you feel like you're ready to move on.

How to tell if you're not ready? Sometimes it's difficult to distinguish between not being ready to move on and just recovering from your last session. If you are unable to complete a session, that's a sign you're not ready to progress. Continue repeating that week until you can comfortably perform the entire workout.

Phase 1: Weeks 1-4 Beginner Level

During the first phase of training, we'll be focusing on technique and good movement patterns. Our intention is to build a strong foundation before moving into the next phase of training. I want you to focus on slow, controlled movement and pay attention to the muscles being worked so we can develop a mind-muscle contraction.

This first phase is also a chance to develop a good routine and enforce healthy habits. One of the reasons why exercise programs aren't always completed is because they're unrealistic and don't fit into your routine. During these first four weeks, we're going to ease our way into training to ensure its sustainability over the next twelve.

Our first phase of training is going to include two workouts. You can choose when you perform these workouts. There are no set days. Whatever fits best into your routine. Ideally, leave two days rest between each workout to ensure you're getting enough recovery between sessions.

Each workout consists of multi-joint, upper body, lower body, core, and mobility exercises. A combination of these exercises ensures you receive a full-body workout.

Week 1 – Day 1:

Total Workout Time: 30 Minutes

Exercise	Reps	Sets	Rest
Air Squats	10-15	2	90 Seconds
Tricep Dips	10-15	2	90 Seconds

Swimmers	10-15	2	90 Seconds
Glute Bridge	10-15	2	90 Seconds
Press Ups	10-15	2	90 Seconds
Dead Bug	10-15	2	90 Seconds
Standing Toe Touches	10-15	2	90 Seconds
Cow	30 seconds	2	90 Seconds

Week 1 – Day 2:

Total Workout Time: 30 Minutes

Exercise	Reps	Sets	Rest
Deadlift	10-15	2	90 Seconds
Bird Dog Plank	10-15	2	90 Seconds
Clams	10-15	2	90 Seconds
Hollow Archs	10-15	2	90 Seconds
Long Lunge	10-15	2	90 Seconds
Hammer Curl	10-15	2	90 Seconds
Calf Raises	10-15	2	90 Seconds
Boat	30 seconds	2	90 Seconds

Week 2 – Day 1:

Total Workout Time: 30 Minutes

Exercise	Reps	Sets	Rest
Plié Squat	10-15	2	90 Seconds
Split Stance Row	10-15	2	90 Seconds
Donkey Kicks	10-15	2	90 Seconds
Leg Raises	10-15	2	90 Seconds
Single Leg Box Squat	10-15	2	90 Seconds
Shoulder Press	10-15	2	90 Seconds
Reverse Lunges	10-15	2	90 Seconds
Sphinx	30 seconds	2	90 Seconds

Week 2 – Day 2:

Total Workout Time: 30 Minutes

Exercise	Reps	Sets	Rest
Single Leg Raise	10-15	2	90 Seconds
Lateral Raises	10-15	2	90 Seconds
Side Lunges	10-15	2	90 Seconds
Cat Cow	10-15	2	90 Seconds
Knee to Elbow Extension	10-15	2	90 Seconds
Shrugs	10-15	2	90 Seconds

Wide Squat	10-15	2	90 Seconds
Cobra	30 seconds	2	90 Seconds

Week 3 – Day 1:

Total Workout Time: 30 Minutes

Exercise	Reps	Sets	Rest
Kneeling Shoulder Press	10-15	2	90 Seconds
Bicep Curl	10-15	2	90 Seconds
Bench Squats	10-15	2	90 Seconds
Bicycle Crunches	10-15	2	90 Seconds
High Knees	10-15	2	90 Seconds
Single Arm Row	10-15	2	90 Seconds
Leg Abduction	10-15	2	90 Seconds
Crescent Lunge	30 seconds	2	90 Seconds

Week 3 – Day 2:

Total Workout Time: 30 Minutes

Exercise	Reps	Sets	Rest
Plank Hops	10-15	2	90 Seconds
Front Raises	10-15	2	90 Seconds
Knee to Chest	10-15	2	90 Seconds

Flutter Kicks	10-15	2	90 Seconds
Mountain Climbers	10-15	2	90 Seconds
Plank Toe Taps	10-15	2	90 Seconds
Jumping Jacks	10-15	2	90 Seconds
Baby Cobra	30 seconds	2	90 Seconds

Week 4 – Day 1:

Total Workout Time: 30 Minutes

Exercise	Reps	Sets	Rest
Lunge and Press	10-15	2	90 Seconds
Press Up Hold	10-15	2	90 Seconds
Wall Assisted Single Leg Toe Touches	10-15	2	90 Seconds
Tuck Ups	10-15	2	90 Seconds
Squat and Press	10-15	2	90 Seconds
Plank Row	10-15	2	90 Seconds
Cossack Squat	10-15	2	90 Seconds
Downward Facing Dog	30 seconds	2	90 Seconds

Week 4 – Day 2:

Total Workout Time: 30 Minutes

Exercise	Reps	Sets	Rest
Weight Hold and Squat	10-15	2	90 Seconds
Single Arm Lateral Raises	10-15	2	90 Seconds
Single Leg Deadlifts	10-15	2	90 Seconds
Hip Lifts	10-15	2	90 Seconds
Plank Jacks	10-15	2	90 Seconds
Curl to External Rotation	10-15	2	90 Seconds
Knee to Chest Box Step Up	10-15	2	90 Seconds
Extended Triangle	30 seconds	2	90 Seconds

Phase 2: Weeks 5-8 Intermediate Level

The second phase of training will prioritize training frequency. You'll notice we've moved from two to three training days a week. The rest between sets has also been reduced to ensure your body is continuing to adapt to more demanding training conditions.

We intend to continue building on our strength gains from phase one while introducing some more advanced movements. Again, I want you to focus on slow, controlled movement and pay attention to the muscles being worked.

During phase two, I want you to continue implementing your daily habits. By now, the honeymoon period of habit building has worn off. Your habits have either been engrained, either you're finding them inconvenient. If it's the latter, cut them back and make them more realistic. For example, if your habit was to walk 10,000 steps per day, but you regularly didn't hit them, cut it back to 6,000. Setting a more realistic target increases your chance of sticking to that habit. Remember, any kind of progress is better than no progress.

Our second phase of training is going to include three workouts. You can choose when you perform these workouts. There are no set days. Whatever fits best into your routine. Ideally, leave two days rest between each workout to ensure you're getting enough recovery between sessions.

Each workout consists of multi-joint, upper body, lower body, core, and mobility exercises. A combination of these exercises ensures you receive a full-body workout.

Week 5 – Day 1:

Total Workout Time: 27 Minutes

Exercise	Reps	Sets	Rest
Lunge Jumps	10-15	2	75 Seconds
Plank Toe Taps	10-15	2	75 Seconds
Reverse Lunges	10-15	2	75 Seconds
Alternating Knee Touches	10-15	2	75 Seconds
Mountain Climbers	10-15	2	75 Seconds
Tricep Dips	10-15	2	75 Seconds
Single Leg Deadlifts	10-15	2	75 Seconds
Dynamic Pigeon	45 seconds	2	75 Seconds

Week 5 – Day 2:

Total Workout Time: 27 Minutes

Exercise	Reps	Sets	Rest
V-Ups	10-15	2	75 Seconds
Deadlift	10-15	2	75 Seconds
Bird Dog Plank	10-15	2	75 Seconds
Clams	10-15	2	75 Seconds
Sprinter Sit Ups	10-15	2	75 Seconds
Air Squats	10-15	2	75 Seconds
Press Up Hold	10-15	2	75 Seconds
Cow	45 seconds	2	75 Seconds

Week 5 – Day 3:

Total Workout Time: 27 Minutes

Exercise	Reps	Sets	Rest
Jumping Jacks	10-15	2	75 Seconds
Plank Hip Dips	10-15	2	75 Seconds
High Knees	10-15	2	75 Seconds
Shoulder Press	10-15	2	75 Seconds
Wide Squat	10-15	2	75 Seconds
Hollow Archs	10-15	2	75 Seconds
Tricep Dips	10-15	2	75 Seconds
Hero	45 seconds	2	75 Seconds

Week 6 – Day 1:

Total Workout Time: 27 Minutes

Exercise	Reps	Sets	Rest
Swimmers	10-15	2	75 Seconds
Wall Assisted Single Leg Toe Touches	10-15	2	75 Seconds
Hip Lifts	10-15	2	75 Seconds
Plank Hops	10-15	2	75 Seconds
Single Arm Row	10-15	2	75 Seconds
Knee to Chest Box Step Up	10-15	2	75 Seconds
Long Lunge	10-15	2	75 Seconds
Pigeon	45 seconds	2	75 Seconds

Week 6 – Day 2:

Total Workout Time: 27 Minutes

Exercise	Reps	Sets	Rest
Bicep Curl	10-15	2	75 Seconds
Standing Toe Touches	10-15	2	75 Seconds
Flutter Kicks	10-15	2	75 Seconds
Single Leg Box Squat	10-15	2	75 Seconds
Shrugs	10-15	2	75 Seconds
Weighted Lunges	10-15	2	75 Seconds
Bicycle Crunches	10-15	2	75 Seconds
Extended Triangle	45 seconds	2	75 Seconds

Week 6 – Day 3:

Total Workout Time: 27 Minutes

Exercise	Reps	Sets	Rest
Plank Row	10-15	2	75 Seconds
Glute Bridge	10-15	2	75 Seconds
Side Plank	45 seconds	2	75 Seconds
Single Leg Raise	10-15	2	75 Seconds
Lateral Raises	10-15	2	75 Seconds
Donkey Kicks	10-15	2	75 Seconds
Leg Raises	10-15	2	75 Seconds

Kneeling Prayer	45 seconds	2	75 Seconds

Week 7 – Day 1:

Total Workout Time: 27 Minutes

Exercise	Reps	Sets	Rest
Lunge and Press	10-15	2	75 Seconds
Split Stance Row	10-15	2	75 Seconds
Bench Squats	10-15	2	75 Seconds
Low Plank Knee to Floor	10-15	2	75 Seconds
Knee to Elbow Extension	10-15	2	75 Seconds
Inverted Push Up	10-15	2	75 Seconds
Knee to Chest	10-15	2	75 Seconds
Crescent Lunge	45 seconds	2	75 Seconds

Week 7 – Day 2:

Total Workout Time: 27 Minutes

Exercise	Reps	Sets	Rest
Roll Outs	10-15	2	75 Seconds
Kneeling Shoulder Press	10-15	2	75 Seconds
Hammer Curl	10-15	2	75 Seconds

Single Leg Deadlifts	10-15	2	75 Seconds
Tuck Ups	10-15	2	75 Seconds
Burpees	10-15	2	75 Seconds
Press Up	10-15	2	75 Seconds
Cobra	45 seconds	2	75 Seconds

Week 7 – Day 3:

Total Workout Time: 27 Minutes

Exercise	Reps	Sets	Rest
Side Lunges	10-15	2	75 Seconds
Cat Cow	10-15	2	75 Seconds
Russian Twists	10-15	2	75 Seconds
Front Raises	10-15	2	75 Seconds
Weighted Squats	10-15	2	75 Seconds
Plank Tucks	10-15	2	75 Seconds
Weight Hold and Squat	10-15	2	75 Seconds
Round Forward Fold	45 seconds	2	75 Seconds

Week 8 – Day 1:

Total Workout Time: 27 Minutes

Exercise	Reps	Sets	Rest
Plank Raises	10-15	2	75 Seconds
Cossack Squat	10-15	2	75 Seconds

Leg Raise with Clap	10-15	2	75 Seconds
Squat and Press	10-15	2	75 Seconds
Front to Lateral Raises	10-15	2	75 Seconds
Bulgarian Split Squats	10-15	2	75 Seconds
Plank Rotation	10-15	2	75 Seconds
Baby Cobra	45 seconds	2	75 Seconds

Week 8 – Day 2:

Total Workout Time: 27 Minutes

Exercise	Reps	Sets	Rest
Jumping Lunges	10-15	2	75 Seconds
Curl to External Rotation	10-15	2	75 Seconds
Leg Abduction	10-15	2	75 Seconds
Alternating Superman	10-15	2	75 Seconds
Squat Jumps	10-15	2	75 Seconds
Single Leg Raise	10-15	2	75 Seconds
Calf Raises	10-15	2	75 Seconds
Camel	45 seconds	2	75 Seconds

Week 8 – Day 3:

Total Workout Time: 27 Minutes

Exercise	Reps	Sets	Rest
Dead Bug	10-15	2	75 Seconds
Inverted Push Up	10-15	2	75 Seconds
Donkey Kicks	10-15	2	75 Seconds
Air Squats	10-15	2	75 Seconds
Bicep Curl	10-15	2	75 Seconds
Clams	10-15	2	75 Seconds
V-Ups	10-15	2	75 Seconds
Glute Bridge	45 seconds	2	75 Seconds

Phase 3: Weeks 9-12: Advanced Level

The third phase of training will prioritize strength. You'll notice we've reduced the rest time and increased the number of sets. Again, this is to ensure your body is continuing to adapt to harder training conditions.

We intend to continue building on our strength gains from phases one and two while introducing more weight. Still focus on slow controlled movements, but now your muscles are more adapted to them, we can add more weight and tension.

I want you to continue implementing your daily habits during phase three and add new ones if your old ones are now second nature. If you're still struggling, scale them back until you can find an achievable target.

Our third phase of training is going to include three workouts. You can choose when you perform these workouts. There are no set days. Whatever fits best into your routine. Ideally, leave two days rest between each workout to ensure you're getting enough recovery between sessions.

Each workout consists of multi-joint, upper body, lower body, core, and mobility exercises. A combination of these exercises ensures you receive a full-body workout.

Week 9 – Day 1:

Total Workout Time: 40 Minutes

Exercise	Reps	Sets	Rest
Burpees	10-15	3	60 Seconds
Split Stance Row	10-15	3	60 Seconds

Jumping Jacks	10-15	3	60 Seconds
Plank Tucks	10-15	3	60 Seconds
Front Raises	10-15	3	60 Seconds
Mountain Climbers	10-15	3	60 Seconds
Side Plank	60 seconds	3	60 Seconds
Standing Forward Bend	60 seconds	3	60 Seconds

Week 9 – Day 2:

Total Workout Time: 40 Minutes

Exercise	Reps	Sets	Rest
Air Squats	10-15	3	60 Seconds
Plank Raises	10-15	3	60 Seconds
Knee to Chest	10-15	3	60 Seconds
Plank Rotation	10-15	3	60 Seconds
Single Leg Box Squat	10-15	3	60 Seconds
Glute Bridge	10-15	3	60 Seconds
Dead Bug	10-15	3	60 Seconds
Superman	60 seconds	3	60 Seconds

Week 9 – Day 3:

Total Workout Time: 40 Minutes

Exercise	Reps	Sets	Rest
Deadlift	10-15	3	60 Seconds

Press Up Hold	10-15	3	60 Seconds
Bench Squats	10-15	3	60 Seconds
Leg Raises	10-15	3	60 Seconds
Lunge and Press	10-15	3	60 Seconds
Bicep Curl	10-15	3	60 Seconds
Hip Lifts	10-15	3	60 Seconds
Boat	60 seconds	3	60 Seconds

Week 10 – Day 1:

Total Workout Time: 40 Minutes

Exercise	Reps	Sets	Rest
Plié Squat	10-15	3	60 Seconds
Tricep Dips	10-15	3	60 Seconds
Clams	10-15	3	60 Seconds
Roll Outs	10-15	3	60 Seconds
Single Leg Raise	10-15	3	60 Seconds
Lateral Raises	10-15	3	60 Seconds
Donkey Kicks	10-15	3	60 Seconds
Downward Facing Dog	60 seconds	3	60 Seconds

Week 10 – Day 2:

Total Workout Time: 40 Minutes

Exercise	Reps	Sets	Rest
Long Lunge	10-15	3	60 Seconds
Single Arm Row	10-15	3	60 Seconds

Bicycle Crunches	10-15	3	60 Seconds
Shrugs	10-15	3	60 Seconds
Wide Squat	10-15	3	60 Seconds
V-Ups	10-15	3	60 Seconds
High Knees	10-15	3	60 Seconds
Plank to Down Dog	60 seconds	3	60 Seconds

<u>Week 10 – Day 3:</u>

Total Workout Time: 40 Minutes

Exercise	Reps	Sets	Rest
Shoulder Press	10-15	3	60 Seconds
Knee to Chest Box Step Up	10-15	3	60 Seconds
Tuck Ups	10-15	3	60 Seconds
Front to Lateral Raises	10-15	3	60 Seconds
Reverse Lunges	10-15	3	60 Seconds
Sprinter Sit Ups	10-15	3	60 Seconds
Hammer Curls	10-15	3	60 Seconds
Reverse Warrior Pose	60 seconds	3	60 Seconds

Week 11 – Day 1:

Total Workout Time: 40 Minutes

Exercise	Reps	Sets	Rest
Plank Jacks	10-15	3	60 Seconds
Calf Raises	10-15	3	60 Seconds
Single Arm Lateral Raises	10-15	3	60 Seconds
Alternating Knee Touches	10-15	3	60 Seconds
Plié Squat	10-15	3	60 Seconds
Press Up	10-15	3	60 Seconds
Side Lunges	10-15	3	60 Seconds
Sphinx	60 seconds	3	60 Seconds

Week 11 – Day 2:

Total Workout Time: 40 Minutes

Exercise	Reps	Sets	Rest
Knee to Elbow Extension	10-15	3	60 Seconds
Weighted Lunges	10-15	3	60 Seconds
Plank Toe Taps	10-15	3	60 Seconds
Flutter Kicks	10-15	3	60 Seconds
Plank Row	10-15	3	60 Seconds
Cossack Squat	10-15	3	60 Seconds
Leg Raise with Clap	10-15	3	60 Seconds

Seated Cat Pose	60 seconds	3	60 Seconds

Week 11 – Day 3:

Total Workout Time: 40 Minutes

Exercise	Reps	Sets	Rest
Jumping Lunges	10-15	3	60 Seconds
Plank Tricep Kickbacks	10-15	3	60 Seconds
Cat Cow	10-15	3	60 Seconds
Single Leg Deadlifts	10-15	3	60 Seconds
Plank Hops	10-15	3	60 Seconds
Weighted Squats	10-15	3	60 Seconds
Hollow Archs	10-15	3	60 Seconds
Pigeon	60 seconds	3	60 Seconds

Week 12 – Day 1:

Total Workout Time: 40 Minutes

Exercise	Reps	Sets	Rest
Bird Dog Plank	10-15	3	60 Seconds
Kneeling Shoulder Press	10-15	3	60 Seconds
Inverted Push Up	10-15	3	60 Seconds

Leg Abduction	10-15	3	60 Seconds
Alternating Superman	10-15	3	60 Seconds
Plank Hip Dips	10-15	3	60 Seconds
Squat Jumps	10-15	3	60 Seconds
Camel	60 seconds	3	60 Seconds

Week 12 – Day 2:

Total Workout Time: 40 Minutes

Exercise	Reps	Sets	Rest
Low Plank Knee to Floor	10-15	3	60 Seconds
Single Leg Deadlifts	10-15	3	60 Seconds
Curl to External Rotation	10-15	3	60 Seconds
Shrugs	10-15	3	60 Seconds
Weight Hold and Squat	10-15	3	60 Seconds
V-Ups	10-15	3	60 Seconds
Bulgarian Split Squats	10-15	3	60 Seconds
Hero	60 seconds	3	60 Seconds

Week 12 – Day 3:

Total Workout Time: 40 Minutes

Exercise	Reps	Sets	Rest
Squat and Press	10-15	3	60 Seconds

Wall Assisted Single Leg Toe Touches	10-15	3	60 Seconds
Hammer Curl	10-15	3	60 Seconds
Plank Tucks	10-15	3	60 Seconds
Standing Toe Touches	10-15	3	60 Seconds
Front Raises	10-15	3	60 Seconds
Flutter Kicks	10-15	3	60 Seconds
Standing Forward Bend	60 seconds	3	60 Seconds

Part 5: What's Next?

How To up Your Game

Now the 12-weeks are over, what's next? You want to make changes for life, not just a few months. They've been a good learning process, but how can you continue to progress? Simple, continuously progress your workouts, and keep hitting your daily habits. Real change comes from doing the right things over and over again.

Progression is essential if you want to get stronger. If you keep doing the same thing, your body adapts, and you no longer find it hard. There are a few ways to increase the intensity of your workouts over time:

- Increase the weight
- Increase the tension
- Increase the repetitions
- Increase the sets
- Increase the number of exercises
- Decrease the rest time
- Increase the number of workouts

Throughout the three phases, you steadily made these changes to ensure you progress. You can do the same moving forward. Remember to ensure you have enough recovery between sessions and don't make drastic changes too quickly - you don't want to induce injury.

Conclusion

Throughout this book, you've learned how to live a healthy life through strength training and lifestyle. Let's take a quick recap of the topics we've covered:

Strength training is a type of exercise using resistance to stimulate muscular contraction, build muscle, increase strength, and improve anaerobic capacity.

Various biological changes occur throughout our life span that lead to reductions in muscle mass, strength, and function, also called sarcopenia. The more muscle and strength we lose, the more likely our independence and quality of life will decrease. While we can't reverse or stop the effects of aging on muscle loss, we can delay its progression using exercise, allowing us to live a more independent, high-quality life with less risk of injury.

One of the biggest barriers to exercise is poor motivation and a lack of discipline. We can use a range of methods to strengthen our motivation and discipline, including finding your why, setting goals, being prepared, building healthy habits, and making the journey fun.

In addition to exercise, you should prioritize your sleep, nutrition, and mindset. Focusing on all areas of health will ensure you get the best out of this program.

Each workout should include a multi-joint, upper body, lower body, core, and mobility workout. As you progress, you should continue to increase the difficulty by adding weight, decreasing rest, and/or increasing repetitions, exercises, or sets.

I've given you the tools, and it's now your job to use them. I hope you learned a lot from this book and now feel ready to improve your health!

My kind request

Thank you for your purchase and I hope you enjoyed this book!

Reviews help me tremendously, so your feedback is greatly appreciated, as it lets me know how I am doing!

I can't wait to read your opinion!

References

Fragala, M. S., Cadore, E. L., Dorgo, S., Izquierdo, M., Kraemer, W. J., Peterson, M. D., & Ryan, E. D. (2019). Resistance Training for Older Adults: Position Statement From the National Strength and Conditioning Association. *Journal of strength and conditioning research*, *33*(8), 2019–2052. https://doi.org/10.1519/JSC.0000000000003230

Grandner M. A. (2017). Sleep, Health, and Society. *Sleep medicine clinics*, *12*(1), 1–22. https://doi.org/10.1016/j.jsmc.2016.10.012

Sharma H. (2015). Meditation: Process and effects. *Ayu*, *36*(3), 233–237. https://doi.org/10.4103/0974-8520.182756

Index

Made in the USA
Columbia, SC
29 January 2022

54973227R00146